Look Like a
Winner After 50
with Care, Color and Style

LOOK LIKE A WINNER AFTER 50
WITH CARE, COLOR AND STYLE

by
Jo Peddicord

THE NATIONAL WRITERS PRESS

Produced in the United States of America by
The National Writers Press
1450 South Havana
Aurora, CO 80012

Publisher's Cataloging in Publication Data

Peddicord, Jo
Look like a winner after 50 with care, color and style.
1. Middle-aged women. 2. Health and hygiene.
3. Beauty personal. 4. Color and fashion. 5. Cosmetics. I. Title.
Includes Notes, Bibliography, Index.
(No LC Class. No.)   646.72   94-66013
ISBN 0-88100-082-5   Soft cover
SECOND EDITION
10 9 8 7 6 5 4 3 2 1

Acknowledgements

Production:
Harald Prommel, National Writers Press, Denver, Colorado

Cover Art:
Joyce Hopkins, Hopkins Design Group, Durham, NC

Illustrations:
Paul Koroshetz and **Bobbi Shupe**

Editing:
Lucille Beckstead

Photography:
Michael Edwards, Maxwell Studios, Denver, Colorado
David Monroe, Moxie Studio, Clearwater, Florida

Models:
A.J. Hall, 60, on the cover: Owner/President of Color Images, Inc., Clearwater, Florida, co-owner of Hamilton-Hall Talent Agency, professional actress/model with over thirty years experience, instructor with a nationally franchised modeling agency.

Betty Reed, Denver, Colorado, interviewed in Chapter 5, *Erasing the Wrinkles*, photo on page 68: Professional fashion runway model for over forty years

My sincere appreciation to these caring professionals:
Dr. Linda Fang, Dr. Donald L. Finks, Lois Tschetter Hjelmsted, Dr. George M. Lacy, Dr. Douglas A. McKinnon, Madelyn Stengel, Treva Stutzman

To the courageous women I interviewed for Chapter 10, *Coping with Defeminizing Surgery*, your sincere desire to help women in your circumstances is gratifying and will be remembered.

Jo Peddicord

Dedication

This book is dedicated to women who have spent most of their lives nurturing others in homes, schools, colleges, universities, shops, stores, offices, industries, professions, institutions, and organizations of every kind in every country and who now recognize the need to nurture themselves.

Contents

Introduction

"So much has been said and
sung of beautiful young girls,
why doesn't somebody wake up
to the beauty of old women?"
— Harriet Beecher Stowe,
Uncle Tom's Cabin, 1852.

Looking like a winner after the middle years is possible when we let go of old concepts, embrace new ones, and refuse to be intimidated by the years. It's accepting positive, promising, and recreative concepts to replace the outdated attitudes that say beauty or the winning look is only for younger women.

My "Beauty Beyond 50" makeup classes demonstrate that looking our loveliest is not a matter of youth but of desire and caring.

At one of these classes Jean arrived late and hurried as fast as her cane and body allowed to the last chair. "I need all the help I can get," she panted. Her husband waited in the doorway, saw her settled, then left. Jean looked around at everyone and breathlessly apologized for being late. "I really need some help," she repeated squeezing out a self-conscious smile. There was a ripple of sympathetic chuckling, and the women nodded in agreement. They needed it, too.

Jean had a life-threatening disease that caused a prednisone hump on her back and a fleshy dewlap under the throat. She missed her graceful ballerina figure of many years ago, but she still had a dramatic and impressive face, framed with white curly hair peppered with black. Her large dark eyes flashed intelligently as she concentrated on every word. We talked about the why's and how's of applying makeup –

1

the "trade" secrets that camouflage wrinkles and bring about an ageless attractiveness.

At the end of class Jean asked me for a personal consultation. In her home she learned how to maintain a healthy complexion as well as how to apply makeup artfully. Her husband, who had suggested the class, watched the transformation. Afterwards, he exclaimed, "You look fantastic! Let's go out and celebrate!" That same week she went to a bridge party, and for the first time in years was complimented on how good she looked. She not only looked lovely, she felt lovelier.

Too often we consciously or unconsciously associate beauty with youth, but true beauty is ageless. Once we accept that, it is natural and appropriate to look as good as we want to.

Many women never think of themselves as attractive. Sometimes they have been put down so subtly and convincingly that they unconsciously accept themselves as unattractive instead of challenging a derogatory remark, or considering it mistaken. Too often we accept critical opinions without questioning them.

"Why all this fuss about beauty or glamour?" critics ask. Granted appearance should never be more important than what we say or do, but this is a visual society. Beauty is important. It's pleasant, soothing to the senses and inspires joy. That's why we enjoy gardens, hike in the mountains, walk in the park, listen to concerts, browse through art museums, hang pictures in our homes.

Dr. Maxwell Maltz[1], a plastic surgeon, writes in his book, *Psycho-Cybernetics*, that self-esteem is as necessary to the spirit, as food is to the body. For this reason, beauty, glamour, style, whatever you want to call it is essential to the maturing years. When a woman creates her best appearance, this helps her to overcome some of the loneliness and rejection she may feel with advancing years.

Most societies see the etched face on men as masculine, even macho; but on women, it's "old." This is beginning to change. Care and makeup take years off the face and replace "old" with "ageless." When this happens, we have a better sense of well-being.

An over-60 woman said she had little need for makeup since she wasn't dating anymore. This harps back to teen age years when a date was THE most important event. Glamour is much more than a means to attract romance. It's a practical, personal necessity that enhances what nature gave us and shows a wholesome respect for the person we are. When you look in the mirror and think, "Not bad! You look pretty good even if I do say so," you walk taller with a happier step. That's the whole idea. Our best look gives us a better self-concept and the edge in career pursuits, personal relationships, all activities.

A nurse in a large metropolitan hospital said the way she looked had an effect on her patients. When she had a caring appearance, they were cooperative and cheerful. When she looked ordinary, they complained and acted cantankerous. A similar message came from a school teacher who said when she wore makeup, she had fewer disciplinary problems. Rightly or wrongly, the patients and students sensed that the nurse and teacher cared more about them when their appearance was better than "ordinary."

EVERYONE enjoys seeing a lovely woman. One Sunday morning my seventy-plus mother was leaving her home as a young man walked by. He glanced at her and suddenly stopped to say, "My, you look lovely this morning!" Mother was astounded. No one had told her she looked "lovely" since father died many years ago. This compliment from a stranger brightened her whole day. Until then, she had been too focused on the wrinkles and plumpness to recognize her ageless beauty.

Kaylan Pickford says in her book, *Always Beautiful,* that the advertising media conditions us to believe there is only one age that women are beautiful. According to them, our golden age began in the teens and ended at 30.

The United States' 1984 census figures indicate women over 45 constitute more than one-third of the female population. At this time publications on fashion and glamour have comparatively little information for women in this group. Fashion catalogues and brochures feature young women in mature-looking clothing, flattering neither the model nor the clothes. Looking at fashion show audiences, we see they are primarily women over forty-five. It's no wonder they enthusiastically applaud their peers who are models.

Close to 100 percent of the women over 40 wear eye glasses of some kind. How many times have you seen women past the middle years in these advertisements? Even magazines geared to the fifty-plus market do not have fifty-plus women in their optical wear ads. Fortunately, with each passing year the fashion and cosmetic industries are improving their focus and recognizing where the majority of the market is and what our needs are.

Some department stores are actively addressing the fifty-plus population. Carson's full-page advertisement in a Chicago newspaper featured an over-fifty model wearing lingerie with the words "beauty is timeless."

On the other hand, maybe the industry has mirrored our acceptance of mediocrity. Many women have been reticent about a spiffy appearance that says "fun." Has the absence of advertisements that feature beautiful mature women brainwashed us into thinking that glamour is not for us? It's taken us years to develop a special inner beauty. It's now time to encourage that beauty to be manifested outwardly as well.

Using only 15 percent of the information in this book will help you select suitable fashions, hair styles and makeup that do just that. This attractive new look will boost morale and bring about a more positive outlook. The positive feeling is crucial. Sometimes we have to struggle to hold on to it, but once we discover its importance, we will never surrender to negativity.

Julie Davis in *The Allure Book*[3] writes, "Thinking positively is step one. Projecting this positive energy through body language is step two. This means acting confident even if you don't yet feel it: head held high, shoulders straight, eyes interested. If you don't believe in the power of having an aura of confidence, take a walk along any busy avenue. Look at the faces of the people around you. Those who are smiling and projecting positive feelings are attractive. Those who have unpleasant expressions and downcast postures make you look the other way."

If you were content in the negative nest of "I can't," or "I'm not," you wouldn't be reading this book. Chances are you've been nurturing people most of your life. There's nothing wrong with that, but now let's expand your caring. It's time to nurture you.

> Looking your best not only helps you to keep a positive outlook but also encourages others.

1

The Magic of Color

"Color enriches the world and
our perception of it; a colorless
world is almost unimaginable."
— *Color* by Marshall Edition Ltd.[1]

Color is as important to ageless beauty as the sun is to earth. It makes us look younger or older, heavier or thinner, lovely or dowdy and magnifies inner beauty.

At the beginning of a makeup class, two women complained about the rude treatment they had received in a restaurant.

"Why, I was treated as a non-person!"

"Yes, that happened to me, too," the other one chimed in.

"How did you look that day?" I asked.

"Oh, just about the way I do now, I guess."

"Did you smile when you were talking to the waiter?"

"Well, I don't know. Probably not. I haven't been feeling very well lately. What difference does that make?"

"All the difference in the world. When you look your best and smile, people treat you better."

What people see tells them a lot about the person you are, and color plays a quiet but dynamic role in forming that impression. Another influence, our smile, colors the personality just as effectively as the hues in the rainbow color the body. The combination of an attractive, colorful appearance and a smile says, "I care. I care about you, and I care about me."

In early 1987, a color photo of Helen Hayes appeared on the front page of *USA Today*. She looked very much her regal self, but without the soft facial colorings and her smile, she would have faded into the newsprint. Unless we utilize the magic of color that transforms a plain look into one with vitality, we fade into the landscape. The Pygmalion and My Fair Lady stories are not far-fetched. They have enduring significance.

Throughout history outstanding women have ingeniously combined stunning colors with fashion and cosmetics. Over twenty centuries ago Cleopatra's high style and makeup—the dramatically defined eyes—left an indelible impression that still lives on.

Her glamour was amplified by Elizabeth I, who ruled England from her twenties to her seventies. Elegant coiffures, makeup, jewels, and vibrant colors in gem-studded gowns contributed to Her Majesty's undisputed superiority in the 1500s. Her dynamic presence impressed her court and the crowds with her undisputed authority and poise. Even when she was dying, a biographer relates she was fully clothed with makeup; she was that concerned about image.

The Psychology of Color

Johannes Itten wrote in *The Art of Color*, "Colors are forces, radiant energies that affect us positively or negatively, whether we are aware of it or not."[2] These color forces vibrate warmth, energy, tranquility, and their opposites, which, in turn, affect health, comfort, happiness and safety.[3] Since yellow is the most luminous color in the spectrum, has the highest visibility, and is conspicuous under all lighting conditions, it is used in over 20 traffic signs including STOP.

The psychological capacity of color to affect human behavior has been proven by extensive research. From industrial, government, and armed services facilities to hospitals, schools, and businesses—people react to the cheery or drab color combinations in their environment.

"We do know that people feel happier when surrounded by certain colors," *The Standard Textbook for Professional Estheticians** states. "Some color experts say that the colors we use in our homes are definite indications of personality traits. For example, people who surround themselves with cool colors such as green and blue may be expressing their desire for peace and tranquility. People who use an abundance of bright colors such as red, orange, and yellow are usually people who love gaiety and are outgoing...

"We may not realize to what extent we are affected by color, but when you awaken on a dull, gloomy morning, you probably will reach for something bright and cheerful to wear."[4]

When you are feeling aches and pains, that is the time to wear bright, lively color, because the body responds to colors that suggest vitality. The psychological healing power of color is a major consideration in the interior decoration of hospitals and care facilities. Color-healing, an ancient science, is described in Faber Birren's book *Color Psychology and Color Therapy*. Mr. Birren's research and professional consultation worldwide in color science is extensive and impressive.

People with color allergies feel a definite discomfort and dislike for certain colors. During the brief color analysis of each person in our makeup classes, the color that gets the most negative response is orange. Some women physically withdraw from it. Only a small percentage like or look good in orange. The favorites are red, misty green and peach.

---

* Reprinted by permission of Milady Publishing Company from the publication, *Standard Textbook for Professional Estheticians*, by Joel Gerson.

Colors cause emotional responses. Certain ones "feel" comfortable and others don't. Trust your intuition. Wearing only the colors that kindle confidence and brighten your countenance is advantageous. When you wear colors that attract compliments, you can't help feeling happier.

Be adventurous and try different colors. It's exciting to find a new shade that is positively smashing. Perhaps we never thought of wearing it, or maybe we wore it 30 years ago and now have the nonsensical idea we are too old for it. If it beautifies, wear it.

The Color Personality_____

Each of us has a distinctive color personality composed of all the shades in the rainbow, but in a one-of-a-kind combination. Examine the many shades in your skin, hair and eyes. These plus their relating and complementary colors constitute your color personality and are your best choices for any item placed on your body and in your environment.

Regardless of ethnicity, the skin contains the three primary colors—yellow, red and blue. Everyone's skin has yellow plus melanin, the darkening agent. The red and blue blood supply bring in the other two primary colors. These physiological elements create a predominance of either a blue or yellow coloring element in the pigmentation.

> The undertones created by the predominance of blue relate to cool colors, made from a dominant blue base.

> The undertones created by the predominance of yellow relate to warm colors, made from a dominant yellow base.

The human race has many complexions. Some of the racial undertones are:

Race	Cool Undertones	Warm Undertones
White	blue-pink	peach-pink
Hispanic, Oriental, Asian	olive	golden
Black	charcoal, ashen gray	golden[5]

The colors that look best on you consist of either warm or cool components.

Color Analysis

Fine, you are probably thinking, but how do I know what colors are warm or cool, and which looks good on me?

The color explosion of the 1980s produced many practical books and thousands of color analysts. Prominent color systems in the United States are:

Color 1 Associates
Joanne Nicholson, President and Founder
2211 Washington Circle NW
Washington, D.C. 20037
Representatives in Canada, Puerto Rico, France, Philippines, Germany, Indonesia, Singapore, Australia, Bangladesh, Israel, Japan, Tunesia

Color Me A Season
Bernice Kentner, Founder
Dean Kentner, President
1070 Shary Circle
Concord, CA 94518-2491
Representatives in Canada, Mexico, Panama, East and West Germany, Great Britain, France, Italy, Norway, Sweden, Australia, Hong Kong

A color analysis by a qualified professional is worth the time and money especially if color has always been a problem. In some women the physiological difference between the warm and cool undertones is borderline, causing color confusion. This is eliminated by a qualified analyst.

Besides being fun and educational, a color sitting opens the mind to a broad range of enticing, new shades. The client is given fans, booklets or folders suitable for the individual, containing anywhere from 20 to 200 shades. These are excellent time savers when you are shopping for clothes, makeup, household decorations and furnishings, anything pertaining to color.

Ethically, a good color analyst should guarantee satisfaction. If you have had an analysis and don't feel right about the recommended colors, something is wrong. In the case of dissatisfaction, the analyst should offer another session to resolve the question, or refund the cost and refer the client to another analyst.

Do Your Own Color Analysis

Some cosmetics companies color code their products with simple tests to identify whether the customer is "warm" or "cool" which can be helpful. You can also:

- Apply two shades of foundation or base (at a cosmetics counter), one with a blue base (cool) i.e. rose or natural beige and one with a yellow base (warm) i.e. golden beige. Place it where you have no makeup or the inside of your wrist. The shade that blends naturally with your skin is the right one. If you have difficulty deciding under store lights, compare the shades in daylight.

- Browse around a fabric store and find the table with solid red colors. Pick one that is blue red (cool) and one that is Chinese or orange red (warm). If you cannot make this distinction, ask salespeople for their opinion. Then, decide: Does the blue red or orange red cast a pleasing reflection on your face? The right color gives the face clarity; the wrong one makes the face look drawn and older, sometimes even haggard. What is your reaction to each shade? Do you like it?

Seasonal
Color
Systems

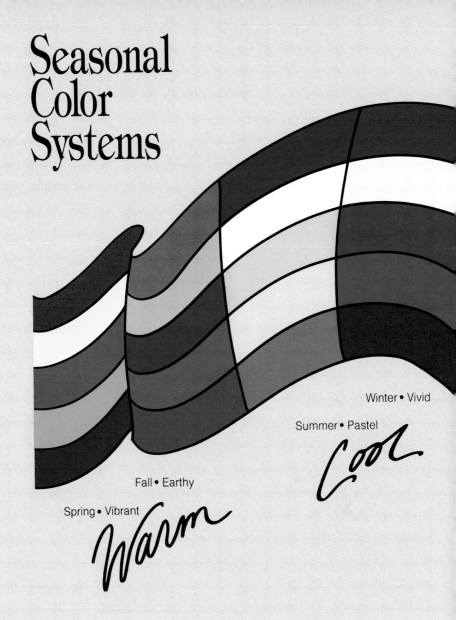

Winter • Vivid

Summer • Pastel

Cool

Fall • Earthy

Spring • Vibrant

Warm

• The warm and cool of five colors •

- If a mirror is not handy, some women have successfully made a color decision by draping the fabrics on the lower half of their arms and noticing the ones that look best against the skin.

While you are in the fabric store, observe the difference in shades of black—the flat black (cool) versus the richer (warm) black; the stark white (cool) versus the creamy (warm) white. Then, use this comparison with other fabric colors. Blues, purples, black and white can be formulated with either a dominant blue or yellow under base. Observing this difference helps to train your eye.

Our intuitive preference is also a strong indicator. Examine the clothing in your closet. If you see lots of pastels or deep, jewel tones, this shows a preference for cool shades. If there are bright, vibrant or earthy colors, this favors the warm ones.

Your most flattering shades are either in the warm dominant or cool dominant family of colors. Some people wear shades from both temperatures as well as gold and silver jewelry together. Even here, their most flattering metals are either cool or warm, gold (warm) or silver (cool).

Color and Makeup

No matter how well it is applied, makeup is not natural-looking and professional if the colors are wrong. Before discussing application in makeup classes, we analyze each woman's color personality, using both warm and cool shades in two or three color groups such as the reds, purples, and greens. Under the chin of each person we hold a warm and cool shade in the same color family. Someone will say, "That color turns her face grey." We'll try the opposite temperature, and they will remark, "Yes, that lightens up her face and she looks much better." When someone is draped with a color she dislikes, many times she will shake head and say, "Oh, no, I don't like that one bit!

Comparing yellow-based and blue-based colors with the complexion is decisive. Your individual rainbow of colors minimizes the lines and shadows, clarifying the complexion. The wrong colors accentuate shadows or blotches and make the skin look pale, sallow or dull.

Select makeup according to your skin. For example, if your undertones are cool, you want lip color and blush shades related to the orchids, roses, mauves, or blue-reds. If they are warm, look at the corals, apricots, bronzes, or orange-reds. Some cosmetics manufacturers color code their products as warm or cool.

Because the cells that produce pigmentation decrease as we age, the skin gets paler, and this is why makeup is more important after thirty.

Linda, one of the women in a makeup class, had a flawless, colorless complexion with Grecian contours. The beauty potential was so apparent that women couldn't help asking her why she didn't wear makeup. She responded, "I don't know how, and I'm afraid of looking unnatural."

Starting with foundation, she learned by applying soft colorings feature-by-feature, each step unveiling her true loveliness. When we finished, she was amazed at the beautiful woman who smiled back in the mirror. She never thought of herself as attractive, and the transformation was almost more than she could believe. Her face before and after the makeup was like comparing a flower garden in a black and white photo with one in color.

When you are uncertain as to which eye shadow, blush or lip color to wear, hold them on the garments to see if they harmonize. If accessories have color prominence, match your cosmetics to them. It's fun to mix makeup colors to get new shades.

Color and Clothing

Color is almost more important than style. Unconsciously, we won't wear even a stunning designer fashion if it's the wrong color. It just hangs around and never goes out, making us wonder why we never wear it. Consequently, we save time when we shop first by color, then style.

The colors around the throat and shoulders reflect up to the face. So, these colors should be your best light or bright shades. Be careful about wearing dark colors like navy and black around the face. They bring out the facial shadows caused by wrinkles or lines. One way to soften this effect is to tuck a chiffon or silk scarf with white-infused pastels into the V-neck or jewel neckline of a suit or dress in the dark hues.

Using monochromatic (shades in same family) colors in an outfit such as a pink blouse with a darker shade of pink in the slacks is figure-friendly and pleasing to the eye. Bold colors look best with neutrals, for example, a fuschia, red or cobalt blue sweater over a white linen skirt. The most common neutral colors are white, gray, beige, brown, navy and black.

Brilliant colors belong in our wardrobe when they fit our personality and comfort zone. An Italian-born grandmother said she was so happy to live in the United States. In Italy she would be expected to wear the dark blues and blacks that are traditionally proper for women past forty. Here, she can wear the brighter shades that make her feel alive.

Total Color Harmony

Appearance with total color harmony has classic style. Everything works together. This means that all the colors we wear are blue based (cool) or yellow based (warm). For example, if the undertones of your skin are blue, the colors of apparel, cosmetics and accessories are cool. To see how this principle is used, observe the appearance of someone you admire and pictures in fashion magazines.

That Special Color, Red

Red is the most dynamic. It attracts immediate attention and is a primary makeup color. For that reason, it deserves special attention. This high-energy hue is more effective in soft, matte fabrics such as wool gabardine and jersey rather than shiny ones. If you want to soften its exciting impact, combine it with white like a red blazer over a white knit sweater or a white wool skirt.

I attended a Sunday afternoon tea where a woman wore an attractive Chinese red suit, but her lip color was a blue-toned magenta that "pinched" her mouth, blanched out her face, and clashed with the beautiful red in her suit. An orange-red lip color would have softened facial lines and harmonized with the suit. Because red is eye-catching, take care that your cheek and lip colors perfectly match or blend with the red in your clothing.

The Focal Point of Appearance

Since the face is generally accepted as the focal point of the image we present, makeup colorings are no longer superficial but essential to the ageless concept. If the makeup beautifies, the hair color flatters, and you put on a smile, you could wear a burlap bag (the right color, of course) and look great!

2

The Basics

"What is the first thing you notice about a person?" I asked one of my makeup classes. One woman surprised us by saying she noticed a person's tummy first. She appraised people starting at the midsection!

Most of the time the face triggers that important first impression with peripheral vision taking in the rest. The secret of facial attractiveness starts with a cared-for complexion, which is an indispensable base for glamorous colorings.

The life-style habits of many women adversely affect their skin—from health abusers such as the sun, poor eating habits, alcohol, and cigarettes to stress, environment in the workplace, travel, and polluted city air. Because of these and other factors, skin problems are common, making it imperative to nourish and care for the skin with regularity. More and more cosmetic companies are developing excellent skin care products to meet the changing role of women and to give them maximum benefits.

Slow the aging process of the skin by observing the following:

- Use sunscreen when you sunbathe, and keep the face and throat shaded. Excessive sun exposure causes brown spots, weakens the elastic fibers, and damages the underlying collagen. It can also penetrate the thin layer around the eyes, causing pigment changes and dark under-eye circles.

■ To prevent facial tension lines, find stress-relieving outlets such as sports, exercise and/or aromatherapy. (Aromatherapy is the use of essential oils from plants for therapeutic purposes.)

■ Avoid the skin-aging habits of frowning, squinting, scowling, excessive smoking and alcohol. The last two dehydrate and deplete the nutrients in the body. Nicotine constricts blood vessels diminishing the flow of blood to the skin, and inhaling eventually causes deep lines around the lips.[2]

■ Use an effective cleansing routine that includes masking/exfoliating and moisturizing that help to reduce the visibility of lines.

■ Get as much sleep as you require, usually six to eight hours. Lack of sleep shows up on the face.

Before we get into the basics, let's briefly touch on two related components—good eating and exercise. In-depth information on these subjects is available in numerous books and magazines.

Good Eating

Healthier skin is just one of the advantages of good eating patterns. The skin is nourished by nutrients in the bloodstream. A well-balanced diet is insurance for healthy skin. Cut down or eliminate sugar and salt. Eat plenty of fresh fruits and vegetables, nuts, seeds, some fats, and drink as much water as you can. It detoxifies the system by flushing out impurities. Dehydration or lack of moisture in the system is one of the main causes of lines.

Collagen gives the skin resiliency and elasticity. The body's production of new collagen slows down with aging. Oranges are excellent because they are 80% water and contain vitamin C that is essential to collagen production. Vitamin C, one of the least expensive anti-aging remedies, helps to build and maintain collagen and elastin. Various facial products contain collagen because it binds water to the skin's surface.

Certain vitamins are especially beneficial to the skin, hair and nails. These are:

Vitamin A—Eyes, skin, hair, teeth.

Vitamin B_2, riboflavin—Nails, skin and hair.

B complex, niacin—Skin.

B complex, biotin—Hair and skin.

Vitamin E has the strongest healing ability of all vitamins.

Natural Sources

Vitamin A — Dairy products, citrus fruits, green and yellow vegetables, milk, eggs, cheese, cantaloupe, watermelon, apricots.

Vitamin B — Bananas, eggs, yogurt, cheese, nuts, seeds, chicken, potatoes, yeast, whole grains, leafy vegetables, and fish.

Vitamin E — Vegetable oils, fresh vegetables, wheat germ, nuts, legumes, sunflower seeds.

Zinc — Fish, peas, nuts, beans, grains, brewer's yeast, sunflower seeds, dairy products.

Zinc is the most important trace mineral for healthy skin.[3,4]

Cod liver oil, an old cure and a natural source of Vitamins A and D, not only benefits dry skin and hair, but also helps arthritis, strengthens bones, and lubricates all body linings. It is processed in mint, cherry and orange flavors to eliminate the fishy taste. Dale Alexander, recognized for his comprehensive research on the remedial powers of cod liver oil, has lectured extensively and written four books on the subject. In his book, *Dry Skin and Common Sense*,[5] he recommends using one tablespoon of the liquid cod liver oil, not the capsule form, mixed with four ounces of milk or orange juice. Blend with one-half a banana, if desired. For best results, drink it one hour before eating.

Facial Massage and Exercises

Stimulating the skin by gentle massage activates the collagen fibers below the epidermis layer. Wrinkles occur when these fibers lose their flexibility. On a cleansed face, apply an emollient creme or oil. Use the finger pads to gently make continuous one-inch circles over the surface of the face and throat but not the eye area. Try doing this in the shower or bath. The warmth of the steam causes the skin to absorb the moisture that minimizes facial lines.

Constance Schrader in her book *No More Wrinkles*[6] says that facial exercises benefit skin tone and texture, dilating the vascular system and bringing blood, oxygen and nutrients to the skin. Although facial exercises improve circulation of the blood, some critics claim they cause lines and wrinkles. This could happen if the face is not thoroughly lubricated with an emollient creme or oil before exercising or if the exercises are done with jerking movements. The best movement is slow and controlled, building muscle tone and lifting sagging skin. Here are some basic how-to's:

1. Cleanse then lubricate the face. Apply an emollient with the finger pads using upward strokes or small circular motions. Be gentle.

2. Squeeze and expand the muscles in the area you wish to tone and firm up. For example: On the forehead—slowly raise the eyebrows high, then lower them and squint. Release slowly.

3. For the eye area: First apply a moisturizing eye creme.

Open eyes wide and then squeeze them tightly closed. Repeat several times.

4. Devise ways to stretch and relax all areas of your face where you wish to decrease the lines. Do this daily for two weeks and observe results.

5. Blow up balloons to keep cheeks firm, eliminate telltale squirrel pouches and keep the muscles elastic around your lips. Spend a couple minutes each day blowing up a balloon. This also strengthens your lungs.[7]

6. After exercising, hold a teaspoon under medium hot water until the metal is very warm. With the outside bowl of the spoon "iron out" the lines with gentle upward strokes. As the lubricant you applied in step 1 penetrates the skin, think of the lines melting away.

7. Head Rolls. Here's an easy exercise to practice every day. It stimulates circulation to the entire head, eyes, face and neck, keeps throat and jaw line firm and helps to control the development of a double chin. With erect posture either standing or sitting, slowly drop head down, roll to side, back, the other side and down to front. Do slowly three to five times, then roll to the other side three to five times.[8]

Smile!

Contrary to what some people believe, smiling does not cause wrinkles. The opposite is true. Smiling is one of the best exercises to prevent lines. Everything goes up when we smile. Tony Ray, a makeup artist, and Angela Hynes write, "One of the best gravity-beaters is smiling! There is more to it than the mere fact that a happy face has a youthful sparkle. Smiling turns up the corners of your mouth, lifts your cheeks, and crinkles your eyes—all of which counteract the downcast look of sagging muscles."[9]

A smile is also one of our best assets, costing nothing, but saying a lot. Charm in manner as well as appearance is more important now than ever before. Many times we feel, "What is there to smile about?" Dale Carnegie included an entire chapter on smiling in his classic, *How to Win Friends and Influence People.*[10] He describes a smile as therapeutic. Even when you don't feel like smiling, smile anyway, he recommends, not a forced grin but a sincere smile. You need it, and the world needs it.

Smiling creates happiness, good will and the realization that all is not hopeless. Carnegie described a dinner party in New York City where a wealthy woman, who spent a fortune on furs, jewels and gowns but had done nothing about her face, was eagerly trying to make a good impression on everyone. She was unsuccessful because her unsmiling face expressed sourness and selfishness. She didn't realize that what her face said was far more important than what she wore.

"Be cheerful. Keep the corners of your mouth turned up, and hide your worries and disappointments under a smile."[11]

Puffiness Under the Eyes

Eye strain, stress, genetics, respiratory allergies, and too much salt in the diet are some of the causes of under-eye puffiness. Because of the delicacy of skin in the eye area, use products specifically formulated for the eye area and ophthalmologist-tested.

To reduce under-eye swelling, do one of the following during a 15-20 minute relaxation:

1. Place cold compresses such as plastic eye masks filled with cold water or cotton balls soaked in ice water on the eye area. Or, keep two tablespoons in the refrigerator until they are cold. Hold the underside of the spoons on the puffy areas.

2. Try any of these over each puff: one-half slice of cucumber, one-half of a raw fig, or a slice from inside an Idaho potato.

3. Under each eye, place a black tea bag that has steeped for five minutes in a saucer of hot water. Lie down on a towel, press the tea into the skin. After 15 minutes, cleanse.

If you waken in the morning with puffiness, press a cold washcloth on the under-eye area. Cold water is a good toner.

Makeup also helps. Put a pale concealant in the indents under the puffiness and a foundation or concealant, one shade darker than your regular tint, on top of the puffs. Fade out the edges.

Donna Lawson in her book, *Prevention's Guide to Looking Fit and Fabulous at Forty*,[12] writes that some doctors claim bags under the eyes gradually disappear with regular exercise.

> Happiness comes along one smile at a time.

Why Exercise?

Just as constant flow keeps mountain streams pure, so exercise stimulates the flow of blood throughout the body to keep it powerful. The largest organ of the body, the skin, develops a healthy hue and produces more collagen when the body is vigorously exercised. The increased circulation brings more nutrients to the cells and organs and helps retard aging of the skin. The increased oxygen intake also aids the production of new cells.

Many experts believe that half the functional losses between the ages of 30 and 70 can be attributed to lack of exercise.[13] Exercise or any activity that moves and stimulates the body parts wards off heart disease, stroke, brittle and broken bones, and the pain of arthritis. It also improves sleep and

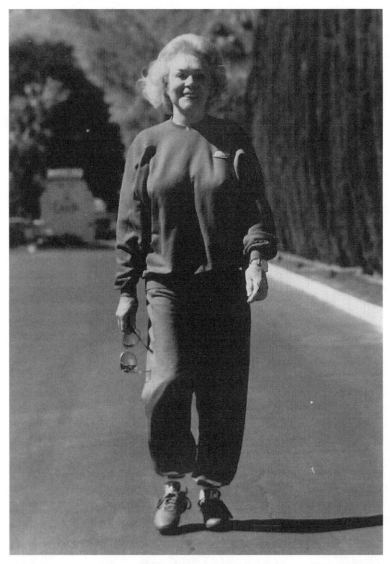

Alice Faye was a film star of the 1930s and 1940s and is wife of bandleader Phil Harris. Now in her seventies, she has been Ambassador for Good Health for Pfizer Pharmaceuticals since 1984. Her book, Growing Older, Staying Young, was published in 1990. She believes, "Once you make exercise a part of your lifestyle, you'll never want to stop . . . one more tip . . . for heaven's sake, have a sense of humor. It really helps you keep your spirits up."

relaxation, lowers cholesterol, and increases flexibility of all joints. The more we put into physical action, the more energy and renewal we get back. Energy begets energy. Benefits are both physical and mental.

Explaining why she didn't exercise, Phyllis Diller quipped she's at an age where her back goes out more than she does![14] If exercise is not for you, find a suitable substitute because the advantages are too great to ignore. A gentle approach to health and rejuvenation, called T'ai Chi Chih, is explained in a book by Justin F. Stone, a former T'ai Chi Ch'uan teacher. The title is *T'ai Chi Chih; Joy Thru Movement*. Through a series of slow, simple movements practiced daily the body and mind are energized and cleansed.

If you feel more critical and grumpy than usual, physical activity will phase out the grouchies. When the physique is exercised and properly fed, not only do the hair, nails, and skin seem to behave better, but attitude improves as well.

This expansive era presents a variety of ways to get the body moving. Besides walking, golf, tennis, skiing and dancing, there are aquasize, swimming, wogging (fast walking), biking, hiking, yoga, weight-lifting, Tai-Chi, gentle aerobics and more. Be aware of relaxing the facial muscles to prevent tension lines. Although running has its advocates, excessive running causes facial skin to droop and other problems. Skin starts to lose elasticity after 30. If you have questions about a suitable routine for you, consult with a physician who understands the value of physical activity.

Ann was in a near fatal automobile accident 20 years ago that crushed both of her knees. After recuperation, she was able to walk without a cane but weakness was always present and her favorite sports, tennis and ice skating, were out of the question. When she was 70, she started lifting weights under the guidance of a teacher who showed her ten steps to strengthen and tone her body. Three times a week she put on her sweats and went to the community center to "pump iron."

After regularly pushing weights with her legs she became more sure-footed than at any time since the accident. Her attitude took a happy turn, energy increased and feelings of well-being blossomed.

At the summer Senior Games in Greeley, Colorado men and women from 55 to over 80 play tennis, swim, throw frisbees, race walk, bowl and bike race to name some of the events. You should have seen the shining faces when they won a medal. Even if they weren't winners, they still pulsed with a *joie de vivre*, basking in the satisfaction of team play and meeting other gutsy people over 55. The non-participants couldn't help but be impressed watching their peers of all shapes and ages, even two sightless swimmers, wrestling with challenges. Many train from one year to the next striving to achieve new goals.

When an over-70 race walker was asked how she maintained her slender figure, she said, "Illness, my dear, illness. I've had about everything wrong with me. Used to dive from the high board. Now I just do ordinary swimming and race walking. Sure do like the race walking. Almost won a medal, too. Maybe next year." And, you can believe she's training for it.

Exercise is as much a part of beauty care as the facial and maybe more. The extra flush of oxygen, the pumping of the heart, the speeding up of the metabolism—all help to rejuvenate the skin and tone the body. Just as important is the mental uplift that erases depression and stress.

Sunscreen

Dr. Thomas B. Fitzpatrick, Chairman of the Department of Dermatology at Harvard Medical School, maintains his anti-aging secrets are "intellectual growth—keeping the mind active, continuing education throughout life, exercise and—perhaps most important of all—moderation in alcohol, food, tobacco, and sun exposure, all primary areas of abuse." He added, "99 percent of premature wrinkling is caused by sun exposure."[15] Over-exposure causes loss of elasticity which results in wrinkles and lines.

As the skin matures, there is a reduction in the epidermal cells that produce melanin, a pigment substance that protects against harmful ultraviolet rays. This changes the skin's immune response, making it more susceptible to sun damage. The skin turns pink where it used to tan.

Every day, twenty minutes before going outside, apply a sunscreen or sunblock. Sunscreens come with Sun Protection Factors (SPF) from two to forty. The higher the number the greater the protection. Use one with an SPF of at least 15, preferably PABA-free, and waterproof if you're going in for sweat or water sports.

The Complexion Care Routine

Skin-priming is the starting point for modern cosmetics, and it pays big dividends. The skin is a sensitive sensory organ, so a complexion care routine is valuable to retain its health and lessen visible aging. There is no guarantee that lines will disappear, but they will lessen. The more consistent and regular you are, the better the results. Think of it as a preserving routine, not a laborious one.

A skin care program also saves time in the application of makeup because the complexion develops an even texture, enabling cosmetics to go on quicker.

Skin-caring involves five steps: cleansing, removing dead surface cells, toning, moisturizing and protecting. If you think that's too much work, keep it simple, but don't neglect it.

Here are a few basic tips:

■ What you do to the face, do to the throat, all around the throat.

- Use upward-moving gentle strokes when cleansing and moisturizing.

- Never roughly push or pull the facial skin.

- Use the ring finger on the fragile area around the eyes.

- Never use hot water. It strips away the protective oil barrier that holds water in.

Cleansing. Conscientious daily cleansing is the secret to an ageless complexion, because it increases the skin's receptivity to moisturizing. An effective cleanser leaves the skin feeling soft and smooth, not greasy or dry. Use the correct product for your skin type and rinse thoroughly—many splashings—with warm water and a washcloth.

If you prefer a bar, look for a non-alkaline, soap-free, facial cleansing product. It rinses easier than soap and is typically milder. Soaps wash away natural surface oils causing dryness and may also leave a chemical residue. A non-soap bar is usually called a beauty or complexion bar without the word "soap" on the label. These products have most of the advantages and few of the disadvantages of soap.

It is not unusual for someone to say that her mother (or grandmother) used soap and water and her complexion was beautiful. According to *The Standard Book for Professional Estheticians,** "Your grandmother may have been one of those people who had a naturally healthy and attractive skin. However, she was not confronted with some of the enemies of the skin that have come about in recent times. Air pollution, chemicals in water, preservatives in food are just a few of the things in our modern environment that may affect the skin. Today it is more important than ever to give the skin proper, daily care."[16]

For dry to normal skin, when you cleanse at night, it is unnecessary to cleanse again in the morning. Just rinse with

---

* Reprinted by permission of Milady Publishing Company from *The Standard Book for Professional Estheticians* by Joel Gerson.

cool water or mist your face. Besides stimulating circulation, cool water constricts the capillaries, invigorating and firming the skin tissue.

Removing the Dead Cells. Skin cells reproduce once a month, sloughing off old cells that are not removed with ordinary cleansing. After 30, the rate of cellular reproduction slows down. The buildup of old, dead cells gives a dull, scaly, uneven texture that magnifies lines and prevents oxygen and moisture from penetrating to live cells underneath. The skin functions better when this buildup is removed by exfoliators, masks, peels or facial brushes.

Jeffrey Bruce and Sherry Cohen write in *About Face* (Putnam Publishing Group), "If you've never exfoliated before (shame!), now you really have no choice. Age brings an accumulation of dead skin cells which, left to their own devices, give a coarse, thick appearance. The dead surface skin must be removed if you're not to look like the alligator lady at the circus . . ."[17]

Exfoliating and masking products contain granules that scrub away useless debris giving the complexion a healthy shine. They do not replace the cleansing process but improve upon it.

Some exfoliants and masks also moisturize. Select one according to your skin type—dry, normal, combination or oily. Exfoliate or mask twice a week for dry skin and three times weekly for oily, either in the morning or evening after cleansing. For combination skin, mask a third time in oily areas only. Massage the product on your face and throat. Do not mask or exfoliate the eye area or places that have signs of breakout or irritation.

Too busy to wait five to ten minutes for the mask? Use the product as a scrub but not "scrub" as in scrubbing the floor! The gentle touch applies. Smooth it on and rinse off. Scrubbing is better than not masking for two or three weeks. Polish the skin with a facial brush to get a similar result.

For a homemade mask try one of the following. Leave it on your face for fifteen to twenty minutes according to your comfort level. Rinse off first with warm water, then cold.

One whipped egg white
One-fourth cup of thick buttermilk
One egg yolk and two tablespoons of honey mixed into a paste
One teaspoon of plain yogurt and one teaspoon of honey, mix
A paste of water and cornmeal or oatmeal.

The best time to mask, exfoliate or apply an alpha hydroxy acid product is on a cleansed face before retiring, not immediately before you put on your foundation.

Alpha Hydroxy Acid Products (AHAs). "Scientific studies have shown that products containing alpha hydroxy acids, when used consistently for a period of time, can improve the appearance of dry wrinkled skin by mild peeling of the surface cells," said Linda Fang, M.D.,[18] dermatologist and developer of the Linda Sy Skin Care System. AHAs do what retin A does, but over longer period of time. It will take more than a couple of weeks to see a difference. A reasonable appraisal takes four to six weeks. The long term benefits are not as predictable as the short term, and the user needs to monitor her skin.

AHAs are made from non-toxic acids found in natural foods. For example:
Glycolic acid is derived from sugar cane.
Lactic acid, from milk.
Malic acid, from apples.
Citric acids, from orange, grapefruit, lemon and lime.
Tartaric acid, from red wine.

Besides removing dead cells, they neutralize free radical damage, soften lines, fade spots and freckles, improve texture, unclog pores, clear up blackheads and whiteheads. AHAs do not prevent aging but sustain healthy, smooth skin. Oily skin requires an oil-free AHA and dry skin, preferably one that moisturizes and is without fragrance or alcohol. Talk to cosmeticians in large drugstores or consultants in skin care centers to get their advice on the best products for your skin. And, ask if you may return it in case it is unsatisfactory.

Follow directions. Regularity is required to maintain good results. For extra sensitive skin, use every other night gradually increasing to every night. Keep out of eyes. If skin feels dry after application, let it penetrate then moisturize. Sometimes a sunscreen is necessary.

Most skin care lines now offer AHA cremes or lotions. Good products are available in drug and grocery stores for under $10. In other stores cost ranges from $10 to $50. The percentage of alpha hydroxy acid in over-the-counter products differs from 1.5% to 15%. If skin is sensitive, start with the lower percentage. Skin care centers and shops have cremes or lotions with 12% and over.

Other uses of alpha hydroxy acid products. The facial AHA product can also be applied to throat and hands. Massage an AHA creme with 8% or more into cuticles to remove dry rough skin. Women with black skin can lighten dark spots caused from breakouts by using an alpha hydroxy acid product or retin-A combined with hydroquinone (a bleaching agent). AHA shampoos help to exfoliate accumulated dead cells that linger on the scalp.

Masking, exfoliating or an AHA is a vitalizing step in your routine if you want a glowing, smooth-textured complexion. Removing the dead cells prepares the skin to be receptive to the next two functions: toning and moisturizing.

Toning. Apply a toner with a cotton ball—moisten if skin is very sensitive—avoiding the eye and lip areas. This step restores the protective acid balance, helps to close the pores (which means a smooth, tighter surface) completes the cleansing process, and seems to "wake up" the skin. Use an astringent like witch hazel for oily areas to absorb excess oil. For dry skin you can use a solution of one-half teaspoon of apple cider vinegar and one cup of water.

Moisturizing. Moisturizers are the key to healthy-looking, comfortable skin. They lubricate, soften fine lines and reduce skin-flaking. Because moisturizers hydrate the membrane, the skin has a dewier "younger" look. Unless you are allergic to collagen, select a moisturizer with *soluble* collagen. Collagen, a protein derivative, "plumps" the skin by holding moisture in and diminishes lines. Phospholipides, complex fat substances such as lecithin found in all living cells, are also waterbinding. Moist skin absorbs better so apply a moisturizer to damp skin.

> Large pores? Mix one egg yolk and same amount of plain yogurt. Let dry on your face for a half hour. Wash off.

Moisturizers should be formulated for your skin type— dry or combination. Apply before the foundation. For oily skin use an oil conditioner. Not only does this priming prevent the foundation from being absorbed into the skin, but the foundation goes on easier. For double benefit, you can mix a moisturizer with a sunscreen of similar consistency. Some moisturizers contain a sunscreen and a tint.

Night-time Treatment. If you use a creme or oil (i.e. vitamin E, cold-pressed avocado or olive oil) after the evening cleansing, be sure it is fully absorbed before going to bed. If it isn't, massage it in around the throat, ears and hands, until greasiness disappears. Do not use heavy cremes or oils around the eyes. Should they get into the eyes, they may cause blurred vision.

Protection. Foundation protects the skin from dehydrating conditions, environmental pollutants and, to a degree, the harmful sun-rays. Some foundations contain an SPF formula.

Each step of a facial care program has its specific purpose

toward maintaining an ageless complexion.

How to Select Skin Savers

1. Ask if you can return the product if you have an adverse reaction or find it is unsatisfactory.

2. Always read the manufacturer's directions.

3. For dry or sensitive skin, look for products that are hypo-allergenic, free of alcohol and fragrance. The words unscented and fragrance-free are used interchangeably. Some products marked as unscented or fragrance-free may still have traces of scent to dull the chemical smell of the ingredients. Look for the words "100% fragrance free."

4. Select products for your skin type:

   - *Dry to normal skin* has small pores and seldom if ever does secretion appear on the surface. Products for dry skin alleviate the dry feeling and restore the skin's optimum moisture balance. Products for normal skin preserve its balance of oil and moisture and help mature skin to have a healthy texture.

   - *Combination skin* may be dry but oil appears on the T-zone (center of forehead, nose and mouth). Products for combination skin control excess oil in the T-zone, leaving dry areas moist and supple and restoring the skin's balance of neither too oily or too dry.

   - *Oily skin* has frequent secretion and large pores. Oil-free products help to control the surface oiliness and to normalize pores.

   - If you have occasional breakout, use oil-free products.

5. Look for the following words that are frequently used in products and in advertisements:

   Collagen—A protein that binds moisture to the skin and gives the skin firmness and elasticity.

Elastin—A protein substance in the skin that gives it firmness and elasticity. Products with collagen and elastin help to control the aging process, smoothing out wrinkles and tightening sagging skin.

Dimethicone—An emollient that helps condition and protect the skin.

Dehydrates—Removes moisture from skin.

Hydrates—Adds moisture.

Rehydrates—Restores normal proportion of moisture to skin.

Emollient—A lubricant which is soothing and softening and may retard the fine lines. Rich cremes have the most emollients.

Exfoliant—An ingredient or product (such as a grainy creme) used to remove the outermost, dead layer of cells.

Humectant—Helps the skin to retain moisture i.e. collagen.

Hypoallergenic or allergy-free—Screened to eliminate all known irritants.

Non-comedogenic—Does not clog pores, or cause blackheads, whiteheads, blemishes.

Occlusive—Seals in moisture.

Stearic acid—A lubricant that relieves dryness by helping to reduce moisture loss.

Syndet—A synthetic detergent; a non-alkaline, soap-free cleansing product. It is milder, more gentle and rinses easier.

6. *Natural Organic Products.* More and more companies are using plants to produce creams, lotions, sun blocks and makeup. The natural beauty product movement is flowering globally, having started in Europe and growing more

popular in the United States. Major companies such as Avon, Revlon, Borghese, Prescriptives, and Lancome have used plant-based products. Clarins and Sisley of France use them exclusively. Some of the "green" beauty companies operating in the United States are Reviva, Aveda, Rachel Perry, and Zia. These products are available in natural food stores and some super markets.

7. Ingredients are listed on the product or the box according to percentage of content with the highest quantity first and the lowest, last. For example, when a product is advertised as having vitamin E or collagen, look to see where it is listed in the labeling of the ingredients to determine how much is in the product. The book, *Face Value* by Zia Wesley-Hosford, includes a dictionary of some cosmetic ingredients and rates them as favorable, unfavorable and questionable. *A Consumer's Dictionary of Cosmetic Ingredients* by Ruth Winter is a reference for description and definition.

8. Cellular renewal and nutritional ingredients seem to rejuvenate the appearance of mature skin. Some of these are: vitamins A and E, panthenol (a vitamin B complex factor), lecithin, shea butter (karite butter), hyaluronic acid, sodium PCA (NaPCA), linoleic acid, shark liver oil, aloe vera extract, jojoba oil, avocado oil, wheat germ oil, gotu kola extract.

9. Skin rejuvenators are exceptional gels or cremes manufactured by all the leading cosmetic companies and many of the smaller ones. They are formulated to turn back the clock on aging skin, revitalizing and giving it a healthier look. In general, they:

   ■ Temporarily minimize fine lines by tightening and firming the skin and reducing puffiness.

   ■ Improve the skin's suppleness by moisturizing within the epidermis.

- Work under the skin to push it out, minimizing lines.

- Restore a youthful glow.

- Shield from sun damage with PABA-free protection.

Centuries ago women had to grind powders and mix compounds in order to concoct cremes, oils and mud packs to preserve their skin, or they accepted as inevitable the aging look. With today's scientific advances, we have products that are easy to use, lightweight, and non-irritating. Physiologically safe products are abundant with even better ones to come.

If the convenience of commercial products is not a factor, why not consider the homemade, money-saving solutions in the book *About Face* (Warner Books), by Dr. Lewis M. Feder, a Board Certified Dermatologist and Cosmetic Surgeon and Jane MacLean Craig, former Public Relations Director for Revlon. The authors detail a routine for each skin type and an appropriate nutritional plan, vitamin therapy and de-aging program. Without reliable information on kitchen ingredients, you could end up using some that clog the pores, or that are too oily or too drying for your skin.

Product Workability

The claims made by cosmetic manufacturers are the results of years of research and hundreds of tests. What a product purports to do means that in the majority of tests, the reactions were as advertised. It may or may not work for you. Everyone's body has a different chemical composition that reacts uniquely to foods, topical treatments and exercise. When a product does not work as advertised, this may indicate that: it conflicts with your body chemistry, you are not using it according to the manufacturer's directions, or the product is defective.

When purchasing a product from a *knowledgeable* salesperson, ask questions until you are fully satisfied about the proper usage. Also ask if you can return it, if it's unsatisfactory.

Reputable companies, conscious of the competition in the marketplace, want customers to be happy with their merchandise, or they are happy to make an adjustment for good will.

The expensive complexes for minimizing lines and wrinkles do not replace or eliminate the necessity of THE BIG FOUR: a daily cleansing routine, good eating habits, drinking plenty of water, and exercise—the modern integration for beauty and health.

Facial Steam Cleaning

Facial steam or vaporizing machines are easy to use and beautify the complexion. They are available from drug stores and beauty supply stores. Carefully follow the manufacturer's instructions. You can also use the "pot" method: Fill a pot with one quart of water, cover, and bring to a boil. Turn off the heat, remove the cover. Place a towel over your head and the pot, creating a tent to catch the steam. Then, lean over the pot eight to 12 inches from the water. Do not put your face too close or you risk burning.

> Night-time nourishment for the face:
> Dab on a pure, unperfumed oil—
> avocado, olive, vitamin E—on driest
> spots. Smooth in with wet fingers.

Procedure. Cleanse first. Protect the delicate areas around the eyes and lips with a light creme. Be sure no emollient is on the rest of your face or throat to block the effectiveness of the mist. Close your eyes during the process. Eye pads are not necessary. Vaporizing helps the lines around the eye area. It only takes five to ten minutes once a week. Allow five minutes or less for dry, sensitive skin. Finalize by rinsing with warm water, or recleansing if necessary. Masking at this point doubles the benefit.

Benefits. This warm diffusion of water on the face and throat:

■ Softens dulling dead surface cells so they are more easily removed;

■ Penetrates the skin, loosening deposits of grease, black-heads, makeup or dirt for a more effective cleaning;

■ Opens pores to eliminate toxins;

■ Increases blood circulation and oxygen because the blood vessels expand;

■ Refreshes, moisturizes and temporarily softens lines. This adds up to a healthier and improved skin tone.

Body Skin Care

Although the skin care steps for the body are the same as for the face, the ingredients in the products may differ because the skin on the face is more delicate than the rest of the body. Body buffing cremes perform the same function as the facial mask, or you can rub away dead surface cells with a soft body brush or loofah, then bathe.

Since water is very important, hydrate your body skin for 10 to 20 minutes by relaxing in a bathtub with one of the following:

A bath gel such as Vitabath, Chicago; Rainbath by Neutrogena, Los Angeles; Orchidee, Roger and Gallet, Paris;
Natural oils;
Half a cup of powdered milk;
The oil from two vitamin E capsules;
One cup of baking soda.

Enhance with a couple drops of a favorite fragrance. While soaking, you can read a book, listen to music, a tape or a radio talk show, snack, peel and eat a juicy orange, sip your favorite drink, or just relax the body and mind. Let the water seep into the skin. This is your personal time.

Pat dry, leaving the skin moist. If you didn't use a bath oil, apply a moisturizer for silky smoothness. With the warmth of the bath, the lotion will blissfully sink into the pores soothing dryness.

Fragrance for Loveliness

Perfumery began as an industry when human development expanded from the agricultural to urban life—about 4,000 years ago. Through millenniums the use of fragrances emitted an elusive influence in religious and devotional ceremonies. Unusual, striking scents were valuable components in healing oils and for incense and adornment. Vials of perfume were buried in the tombs of Tutankhamen, Ramses and other Egyptian kings and queens in order to be convenient for their use in life after death as they believed.

Marc Antony's fate was sealed before he even encountered Cleopatra. The enchantress, clothed in a flowing, diaphanous gown, cruised down the Nile in a vessel with perfumed sails, incense wafting in the breezes surrounding the throne, and her body breathing the most exotic scents.

Fragrance is the ultimate body language. It relaxes and soothes, evokes moods, delights and haunts the mind, and creates a sense of well-being. Some are relaxing to the point of diffusing stress. This sensory perception acts like a time machine conjuring up memories of people and places.

Referred to as bottled magic, scents add a lovely aura to femininity, subtly expressing our distinctive charm and dignity—who we are and what we're like. Because they capture the olfactory sense with a particular message, we need to select aromas to match our personality. Sometimes, scent is as much our identity as fingerprints.

Pick fragrances to fit your moods. For the flirty and feminine, sniff out the florals. For glamour and glitz, go for an oriental or spicy scent. For just plain fun, check out the upbeat, modern fragrances. Selecting an aroma is very personal. Make it an adventure, not a hurried decision.

A unique way to decide upon a perfume, eau de toilette or cologne (listed according to potency) is: Spritz a little on the wrist and taste it. If reasonably pleasant to the palate, it will blend with body chemistry. For more economy, buy refills in the large bottles.

Usually, eau de toilette lasts four to six hours and reaches ten to fifteen feet, while cologne lasts one to four hours and reaches two to eight feet. Alcohol-based fragrance (cologne, eau de parfum or toilette) drops off sharply then remains constant. In some old-line French fragrances, the eau de toilette is weaker than the cologne. If the price doesn't indicate this, the salesperson should know. Oil or creme-based scents (body lotion or bath oil worn as cologne) taper off gradually. Herbal oil fragrances, with citrus and floral bouquets, have good aromatic quality and come in small bottles, easy to carry in the purse.

Fragrance fade-out is a frequent problem especially for dry skin. Here are some solutions:

1. Use oriental, musk, or heady floral scents rather than citrus.

2. If you put fragrance directly on skin, apply a moisturizing lotion first, then the fragrance. The oils in the lotion help to "hold" the aroma.

3. Try an oil based formula—a body lotion, bath or herbal oil—and touch up with perfume or cologne.

Wear it on the pulse points: behind ears, on the inside of wrists and elbows, at the base of the throat or even behind the knees. For lasting power, layer by using talc, cologne or eau de toilette and finishing with perfume. Combine scents whenever you feel like it. If your skin is allergic to fragrance, saturate a cotton ball and tuck in your clothing where it will not irritate the skin, or use an herbal oil fragrance.

When going to bed, even if you are alone, splash on a favorite cologne or dust with scented powder. Why? Because anything that gives a sense of loveliness is good for the psyche, and fragrance on the nightie or the body is certainly that. Pamper yourself with the luxurious feeling of a tranquil aromatic. Marilyn Monroe said she wore Chanel No. 5 to bed and that was about all!

3

Be Your Own Makeup Artist

"There are no ugly women, only
lazy ones."
—Helena Rubinstein[1]

Before a makeup class, I always ask the women why they want to learn about makeup. One woman said, "I'm 81 and think there's so much ugliness in the world that I want to see what can be done about me." During the class we saw how cosmetics took years off her face and beautified everyone. When we finished, there were smiles all around the table.

For centuries women have been fascinated with cosmetics. They are tools for opening the door of opportunity. As mood-altering agents, they change the way we feel about our face, body and even our abilities. They enhance our good features and hide flaws; make us prettier, giving a psychological uplift; and enable us to feel more secure and happier with our appearance. We wear makeup because it boosts self-acceptance and self-confidence.

The cosmetic industry anticipates the current and future requirements of women and develops products whose benefits are physiological as well as aesthetic.

In *About Face* (Putnam Publishing Group) Jeffrey Bruce and Sherry Cohen say, "There is nothing more gorgeous, more appealing, than a ripened woman who has grown accustomed to her face. She isn't trying to compete with starlets when she skillfully brings out the seasoned sensuality she's earned. And the way she does that is with more, not less, makeup—more artfully applied. Because she's fighting gravity and loss of moisture, she has to compensate with better products—and she can't skimp on coverage ... You simply cannot get away with a dab of blush anymore ... I know too many women who spend a fortune on a new pair of boots or a great coat and then walk around with the same, tired, face, because they've been brainwashed to believe that makeup should be drastically reduced after forty."[2]

The Inner Artist

Every woman has an inner artist, an intuitive artistic sense. Look at a woman's appearance or home, and you will see how active the inner artist is in her life. Some women fully express this intuitive perception in the home, garden, handiwork or the arts, but when it comes to their appearance, they turn it off.

Manifestations of the inner artist frequently occur during makeup classes with the placement of colorings. During the discussion of blush, I applied it to Lucy's face and asked her how she liked it. She replied, "It's fine, but I would like it a little closer to my nose." So we blended the color over a degree, and the class agreed they liked it better, too. Although Lucy knew little about makeup techniques, she analyzed, listened to her intuition, and improved her cheek coloring.

Boredom never sets in when we listen to our inner artist for variety in application and color selection. The more we listen to this intuitive artistic sense, the more confidence we have in our face and fashion potential. When this sense is fully actualized, no expert can improve upon its ideas for your beauty.

Key Points _____

Most women know very little about applying makeup. Mary said she went to a department store cosmetic counter to get a little education. The all-knowing salesperson proceeded to apply intense colors without asking her what she liked or preferred. Embarrassed by the vivid shades, which she noticed were similar to what the salesperson was wearing, Mary rushed home, hoping no one she knew would see her— not an uncommon experience.

As you venture into the world of cosmetic artistry, consider the following guidelines:

1. Organize your cosmetics and applicators. Throw out old makeup. Today's products are far superior in content and color.

2. Before you go shopping, think through what you want so you won't be talked into buying something you won't use. Talk to the representative whose face you admire. Test the products if possible. Then, stay in control! Buy only what you like, not what he/she likes.

3. If you have noticeable lines or wrinkles, makeup artists recommend matte, no-shine cosmetics; no oily-looking foundation or blush, iridescent eye shadow or metallic lip colors except where the skin is taut. Shine accentuates lines and wrinkles.

4. Unless your skin tone takes kindly to dynamic colors, look for muted shades. If the colors are intense-looking in the package, use a light touch when applying.

5. If application is relatively new to you, put it on slowly and thoughtfully, until you are sure of your expertise. Don't rush! Carefully blend the colors. If your hand needs steadying, sit down, and place your elbow on the table.

6. Practice the techniques, adapt them to your preference, be creative and have fun. If you make a mistake, so what? Redo until you like it.

7. When you have finished your makeup, check your face by daylight or its equivalent to see that the shades are blended with suitable intensity.

8. Since you need daylight, or quality light for application, you may wish to have your makeup and mirror in a location that has indirect natural light, maybe a dressing table by a window. If this is not possible, find a makeup mirror with lighting controls and use the daylight or "home light" setting. Lighted makeup mirrors are inexpensive and available at discount stores.

9. If it's difficult to see without your glasses, purchase inexpensive magnifying glasses from drug stores or mail order houses. The lenses move up and down on hinges so that you can move one lens down while seeing through the other.

Speaking of mirrors, let's stop being intimidated by them! When you get up in the morning and look at the bland face staring back at you, do you think, "Ugh! Another line," or something similar? Makeup artist Jeffrey Bruce said he saw Sophia Loren without her makeup and "believe me, she doesn't look so hot."[3] There are few women at any age who are gorgeous without makeup.

Everyone in my makeup classes is furnished a mirror and comes with a "bare" cleansed face. As they look in their mirrors, I suggest they get into the habit of thinking, "I'm getting lovelier every day." You should hear the groans! Often someone shakes her head and laments, "I can't say that." But, thinking that phrase, or something similar, is self-reinforcing mental homework, not egotism or pollyannaism. When you put energy and persistence into positive thoughts, even with the lines, wrinkles or bulges, subconscious responses surface to make it a fact.

Tools

Your fingers are often the best tools for blending every thing, even eye shadow.

100% Cotton Balls or Pads. 100% cotton has no abrasives. Anything abrasive such as tissues that contain wood fibers can upset sensitive skin. Cotton balls and pads are used to apply freshener, blend powder blush, remove excess makeup, or dab powder to lips to give the color more staying power.

Cotton, cosmetic, and sponge tips. These may be used for blending eye shadow, removing excess eye makeup, and blending corrective and tinting foundation. The advantage of cosmetic tips is they do not have the fuzz that cotton swabs do. Use them to:

- Soften edges of eye shadow so there are no unnatural lines,

- Edge a line of shadow under lower lashes,

- Erase smudges; dip first in moisturizer, if you wish,

- Touch up the lip line after applying color,

- Cover blemishes; dip in foundation and dab,

- Blend a concealer under eyes where there are dark areas. Sponge tips are excellent to apply eye shadow. Wash sponge tips frequently to maintain cleanliness and purity of color.

Sponges. Damp-dry sponges are useful for an even application of foundation. The edges of triangular sponges may be used the same as cotton tips.

Small Spatula. In order to keep the contents of cremes free of bacteria and impurities from fingers, use the spatula to remove the creme from its jar. Impurities contaminate the product. If you prefer to use creme foundation and do not want a caked on application, use the spatula to pick up a little, mix it with water and then apply. This will result in good but not heavy coverage. A spatula is also handy for mixing shades of creme rouge or lip color. Pick up a little of two shades on the spatula, mix them, and you have a new shade.

Brushes. Brushes come in different sizes for the application of blush, loose powder, lip color, eye shadow and the brows. They are fun to work with. Use the size that is easiest for you. As with sponges, clean regularly with soap and water. You may wish to soak them in alcohol periodically for sanitary reasons. Cleanliness is important because it's possible for bacteria buildup to cause irritation to the skin that you may incorrectly attribute to a product.

Blotters. They are available in 100 percent linen and are very effective for blotting oily areas during the day without disturbing makeup.

The Organizer. To carry cosmetics in your handbag, a plastic bag with a locking top (optional) saves the frustration of digging around to find what you want. It weighs almost nothing and you can see the contents at a glance.

Foundation for the Natural Look _____

Foundation is as important for the natural and/or glamorous look as seams are to a dress. Also called makeup or base, it is indispensable if you want to look unmade-up. With foundation, colorings take on a blended softness that is impossible without it unless you have flawless skin.

Tinting foundation conceals minor imperfections, evens out irregular pigmentation, covers pores and protects the complexion from dehydration, environmental aggressions and ultraviolet rays especially if it has a sun protection factor.

Finding the right shade is often difficult. This was illustrated during a makeup class. We discussed foundation while applying it. As Madeline was putting on hers, the rest of us couldn't help watching. The foundation was actually turning her face a mummy-like grey. When we mentioned this, she groaned and said with exasperation, "I have two bottles of foundation at home that I don't like, and I just bought this today. I never seem to get the right shade." It was even more shocking when she put on lip color because it matched the foundation.

We removed everything and started over with warmer shades in foundation, lip color and blush. These flattering tints brought out her expressive eyes where the others neutralized them.

The problem was the undertones of her skin were yellow while the under base of the foundation and lipstick she purchased was bluish. Evidently, Madeline liked muted colors, but when this foundation with cool tones interacted with her golden undertones, the result was disastrous.

Selecting the correct shade. Some cosmetic companies color code their foundations according to warm, cool or neutral. Choose two or three shades that appeal to you. Place them where you have no makeup—on the jawline, the throat, chest or wrist. In natural indirect light, see how they blend with your skin. One will practically disappear while others look like blobs. The perfect blend is right for you.

Foundation should match the skin on the throat. Too light a shade makes the complexion pasty-looking; too dark emphasizes lines and wrinkles.

BUT, some women with very fair complexions are uncomfortable with a foundation that matches the throat. They think the light shade makes their face look colorless and older. A slightly darker foundation gives a tanned look that is more youthful. Some dark-complected women want a shade lighter than their throat. It softens and brightens the face. In each instance, care should be taken to get the un-madeup look by avoiding too extreme a difference between the tones of the foundation and the throat and by fading out the edges at the sides of the face and under the jawbone.

Creme or Liquid. Creme foundation (often in a compact) is

oil-based and fights dryness, giving a slight sheen, extra lubri-
cation, heavier coverage and protects the skin from
dehydration. Powder/creme foundation provides a non-
shine/matte finish and good coverage.

The liquid or water-based foundation can be used by all
skin types and has a matte finish, unless it contains a moisturizer. A moisturing agent creates a sheen, and for some complexions this is youthful. Coverage is sheerer than the creme
foundation. To cover spots on the face, apply two thin coats, letting it dry between applications, or, use the creme foundation
as an underbase and apply a thin cover of the liquid.

Oily and/or acne-prone skin requires a foundation that is
100 percent oil-free. This product has absorbing ingredients
that reduce oil breakthrough and makeup stays fresher longer.

> A light shade of foundation makes a
> face look wider. A darker one makes it
> look narrower.

For
oily skin, use an oil-free conditioner. If you want the added
protection of a sunscreen, the order of application is: (1) moisturizer, (2) sunscreen and (3) foundation. Some foundations
have moisturizing properties and a sun block. Use only what
your face requires—no more

Application. Pat liquid foundation around the face with
your finger(s) or a cosmetic tip, heavier in the center and less
toward the jaw and the hairline. With a non-absorbent triangular sponge smooth out the color with downward strokes
which cover pores better. The sponge never pushes or pulls the
skin—just glides along the surface—and its corners efficiently
reach into every nook and cranny on the facial plane.

Concealers

Concealers come in different colors and have been around since the 1950s when Max Factor marketed Erace. Today's brands moisturize and also prevent sun damage. Although some are advertised as long-wearing, the most durable are waterproof. They have many uses:

- Fill in tiny lines;

- Lighten dark areas;

- Cover red, brown, age and beauty spots, broken blood vessels, birthmarks and some scars;

- Tone down pink or ruddy pigmentation and lighten bluish areas around the eyes;

- "Bring out" depressions and "recede" fleshiness.

One woman in a class said she was always embarrassed because her throat was red and sometimes people commented on it. When she applied a concealer to this area, she was amazed at the way it neutralized the reddish tone. On another woman, a large brown spot on her cheek magically disappeared when she covered it with a concealer and then her regular foundation. Some women have used lavender powder eye shadow to cover spots and broken vessels.

Pigmentation problems such as scars and birthmarks are more effectively covered by cosmetic correctives which are specifically formulated for this purpose. They also hide varicose veins.

Contouring

Light shades bring out; dark shades recede.

The art of contouring gives the illusion of more or less shape. By carefully blending the edges of the contour color, the effect is subtle, and the technique, invisible. Foundation, concealers, creme or powder blush, even eye shadow offer the possibility of a variety of shadings.

Analyze your face and identify the place you want to redesign. For example:

- If your cheeks are fleshy, place a darker shade below the cheekbones and fade out toward the jawbone with a lighter shade on the upper part of the cheekbones.

- To widen a narrow face, apply blush almost horizontally along the line of the cheekbones toward the ears.

- To "narrow" the broad nose, blend a slightly darker shade of foundation on sides.

- "Shorten" the long nose by blending a darker foundation around the tip and under the nose.

- "Lengthen" the short nose by blending a light or white shade down the middle, carefully blending it into the foundation on the sides.

- For the broad forehead or face, place a darker foundation on sides of the forehead and face. Blend into your regular foundation.

- For depressions like the sides of the temples, hollow cheeks or indents around under-eye bags, use a shade lighter than your skin tone.

The Magic of Makeup

Think of yourself as an artist and your face as the canvas. You're going to create a masterpiece! Don't laugh. You may be pleasantly surprised. During a Glamour for Grandmas class, I asked who wanted to try eye shadow. A woman with creamy white hair said, "Well, I would." Her eyes were sky blue, and she was wearing a matching shirt, so I blended a pastel on the eye lids fading it up to the brows, defined her brows with a blonde pencil, tinted her cheeks with blush and applied pale pink to her lips. I couldn't stop with the shadow because the effect was so exciting. There were "ohs" and "ahs" all around the table. "You look so much younger!" someone exclaimed and others chimed in. I went back to my chair. Looking at her from across the table, I was amazed at the way makeup had actually brightened her hair. It literally glowed. The right facial colorings enlivens not only the face but the hair also.

Do your makeup after deciding what you're going to wear, letting the colors of your makeup and clothing coordinate. An office manager wore a plum lip color and blush every day with all her clothing, whether it was blue, black or red. After a while it was boring to always see the same facial colorings, which frequently clashed with her clothing. Someone probably told her the plum colors were flattering, and no doubt they were with the outfit she was wearing at the time, but not with everything in her closet and certainly not every day!

If you have only one lip color and one blush, it's time to emancipate your glamour box. Using a variety of shades is part of the fun and offers you flexibility to be more creative. Reassess your makeup periodically. Julie Davis says, "New makeup techniques lose their value if the cosmetics you apply aren't up to snuff... If the color is wrong—murky oxblood lipstick instead of a clear red—you won't look as great as you could. Many women will keep using the wrong cosmetics out of force of habit. Take time to evaluate your collection."[4]

Luscious shades pour into the market at the beginning of each season. When in doubt as to which shade to choose, try them on your skin or place them against the apparel you want to match.

Eyes

People like to see eyes. We read each other through the eyes. They tell our story and help us to communicate. In response to the question, What specifically do you want to learn about makeup, the majority of women say eye shadow or something involving the eyes.

The diagram shown in Illustration 1 will help you to identify the parts of the eye as described in applying makeup.

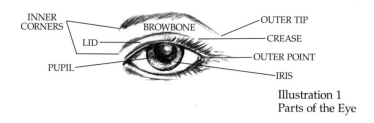

Illustration 1
Parts of the Eye

Brows

Just as a good frame sets off a picture, so sculptured brows set off the eyes. The wrong picture frame can detract even from a masterpiece. Since brows accessorize the eyes, as a frame does a picture, they should be neither insignificant nor overpowering.

Frequently, change is difficult. In one class, a woman with black and white hair had white brows. When we darkened the brows to harmonize with the black in her hair, everyone thought it looked more natural than the white brows and definitely more youthful. But, not her! She was shocked. She had not seen color in her brows for many years and she couldn't accept it now. *Receptivity to change is important if you want the ageless look.*

To find the natural brow line, hold a pencil diagonally from the outer edge of the nose to the outer corner of the eye. The place where the pencil touches the brow bone is the outer point. The inner point is directly over the inner corner of the eye. The natural brow line extends along the brow bone between these two points (see Illustration 2).

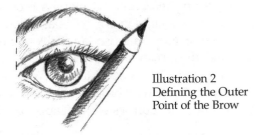

Illustration 2
Defining the Outer
Point of the Brow

The "normal" distance between the eyes equals the width of one eye (see Illustration 3). If the brows are wider from or closer to the nose than "normal" added color balances this as described in the section **Adding Dimension to Special Eye Shapes** on page 65. The highest point on the brows is over the outer rim of the pupil.

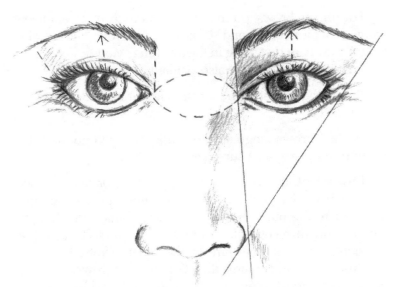

Illustration 3
Defining the Width and
Height of the Brow

Remove stray hairs around the brows to open the area especially when the space between the lids and brows is short.

Sculpturing with Color. Colorless brows are aging. Color that reflects the shades in your hair, as it is now or was, is best. With white or gray hair, use taupe, blonde or slate. The brow pencil and the brush-on brow powder are easy to use. The brush-on powder gives a soft texture. You can also mix colors, for example blonde with brown, or brown with charcoal, or, for a velvety effect dust brows with an appropriate eye shadow.

Thin brows are severe lines that give unnecessary sharpness. They were glamorous on Jean Harlow, but they do nothing for us. With short strokes, add color to make them fuller. The fuller brows add balance to the facial features and are gentler on lines and wrinkles.

Bushy brows are unfeminine. Shape brows by brushing them up, trim the excess length, then brush to the side to see if they are even.

For unruly brows, put hair spray, mousse, or an emollient creme on a tooth brush and stroke over the brows before going to bed and again first thing in the morning. Mousse holds best. Brow control products are also available.

Brows that are straight across without an arch "shorten" the long face.

Arched brows lengthen the round face. Do not arch too much or they take on a surprised look.

Brows that are sparse or too light in color age the face. Darken them. Start with fullness at the inner points and taper the color to the outer points. Exception: Some faces like the long narrow or rectangular require the brows to be as full at the outer points as they are at the inner points. Finish by brushing brows in the same direction the hair grows. Brushing brows is as important as brushing your teeth and hair; it stimulates circulation and encourages healthy growth.

Do not let the inner corners of the brows "hook" under. This is a downward line you do not need. Heighten the color at the inner corners closely paralleling the high point of the arch (see Illustration 4).

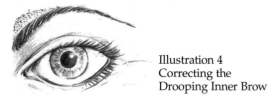

Illustration 4
Correcting the
Drooping Inner Brow

The curve of the brows alters the expression of the face (see Illustration 5).

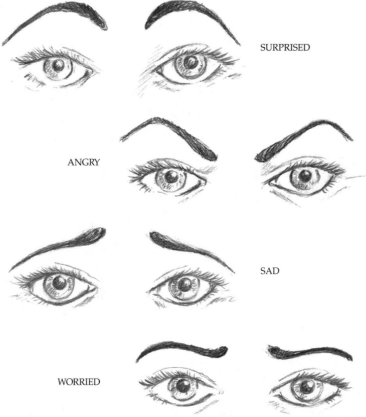

SURPRISED

ANGRY

SAD

WORRIED

Illustration 5

No brows. In one of my classes a woman said every hair on her body left after her last pregnancy three decades ago. She wore an auburn wig that was perfect with her skin coloring. But with no lashes and brows, her eyes had a staring look she didn't like. With a blonde brow pencil that went beautifully with her hair we stroked in color along her brow bone one-quarter of an inch thick at the inner corner decreasing in width to the outer tip. Along her upper and lower lashes we added eye shadow that matched the brows. She was amazed at the normal definition this gave her face and how easy it was to do.

Eye Shadow

To improve the look of shadow, you can get products that temporarily tighten, firm and moisturize the eye area. Shadow adds subtle contour. It comes in pressed powders, cremes, pencils and watercolors. Pressed powders are easy to use. Creme shadows tend to separate into the lines. Applying an eye lid primer or liquid foundation helps to prevent this. Matte, no-shine colors are best for daytime.

When using two or three colors, be sure they blend where they meet. Sometimes we see color from the upper lash line to the crease where it stops. For the more natural look, blend it beyond the crease, fading it out gradually to the brows.

Placement Tips

- Keep an intense shade along lash line.

- Use a pale color to lighten skin tones or shadowy places.

- If you have little contour to your lids, blend a darker shade midway between the upper lid and brow. Fade it up towards the brow line.

- For uplifting, parenthetical shading blend color from center of the lids to the outer corners of the eyes and up to outer edges of the brows (see Illustration 6).

- If the space between the eye and brow is wide, apply an

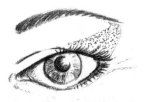

Illustration 6
Uplifting Shadow

earth-tone foundation or beige eye shadow from the crease to the brow, making the area appear narrower.

- If the space between the eye and brow is narrow, apply a pale or light frost or matte shadow from crease to the brow, making the area appear wider.

- *Highlighters.* Iridescent shadows glow. They are very attractive when used correctly. Do not use on crepey skin because they highlight the uneven texture. The best place is directly under the brows where the skin is taught. When placed under a matte shadow, they have a lower intensity.

- For a tinge of color place blush on the brow bone.

Guidelines for Selecting Eye Shadow Colors. Shadow colors outnumber all other cosmetic colors because the jewel tones of the iris are accentuated by a wide spectrum of tints. Select colors to harmonize with your skin tone and sometimes, but not necessarily always, your outfit.

Choosing the same color as your eyes dulls the iris.

Brown shadow is flattering to almost every skin tone. Avoid blue or purple if they accentuate under-eye veins.

Aqua or lavender is good for almost everyone and plays down yellow undertones.

Light colors such as pale pink and peach make eyes appear larger, more open. Dark colors close them in and accent lines.

If you can't decide on a color, barely blend on a concealer.

Here are some more suggestions:

If your irises are: Select

Brown	Mauve, olive, plum, camel, taupe, green
Brown/black	Taupe, grey, olive, mauve, dark green or dark brown
Blue	Grey, mauve, sand, plum, navy, rose
Green	Camel, taupe, turquoise, orchid
Hazel	Grey, heather, olive, camel, cocoa, apricot, peach, dark green
Violet	Taupe, olive, mauve, dark green

At cosmetics counters, try out the shades on the back of your hand or inside wrist.

> Blue, green, or purple eye shadows
> are seldom subtle or natural-looking.

Lashes

Lashes with color and curl look longer. Beauty salons dye lashes with color that lasts eight to ten weeks.

Mascara thickens, conditions and adds color. Pumping the wand up and down sucks air into the tube, drying out the product. Just swirl the wand around, then remove.

Bacteria easily builds up in the tube and can cause infection. For this reason, consider replacing it every three to six months to eliminate any possibility of infection. Reactions are not common, but why risk it? If your mascara stings, try the hypoallergenic brands and always ask whether or not you can return the product if you have a problem.

Applying Mascara. Stroke on from roots to tips. To catch the tips, hold the wand vertical to the upper lashes and brush across, then straighten from roots to tips. For the lower lashes, hold the wand horizontal, brush across tips, then straighten (see Illustration 7).

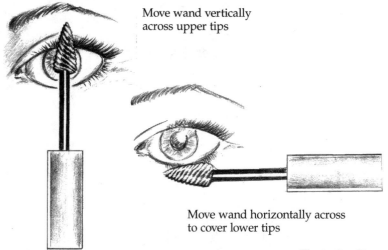

Move wand vertically across upper tips

Move wand horizontally across to cover lower tips

Illustration 7

After mascara dries, remove any clumping by separating the lashes. Use a lash comb, a small brush, or an old, clean mascara wand. To protect against flaking below the eyes, blot lashes with a tissue.

Lash curlers are popular, and so is the spoon method of crimping the lashes. Here's how it works:

- Hold a teaspoon under hot water till warm and dry off.

- Place spoon in your hand with the thumb inside the concave bowl.

- Hold spoon so lashes are between thumb and concave bowl.

Press and curl up as if you were curling a ribbon. One side takes more maneuvering than the other, but practice makes it easy.

> Even when you don't wear mascara, curl your lashes for the bigger, open-eyed look.

Extra lashes are very attractive and a good alternative when lashes are short or thin. Women who use them regularly find they are as easy to put on as lipstick. Placed at the outside corners they give an alluring lift. Be sure to trim to a natural-looking length.

Lining the Eyes

Lining eliminates the nondescript look, especially if you wear glasses.

For a clear, refined line, use the eye lining pen with a fine point. As compared to the pencil eye liner, it is less likely to blur if your eyes water. If you want more softness, smudge the line with a sponge tip.

Pencil liners come in a few colors with brown and black being the most popular. A navy blue liner makes the whites of the eyes whiter, but blue in any eye product draws attention to blue coloration in the eye area. Pen liners come in brown and black.

Application. Open your mouth slightly to relax the face. If you need more steadiness, rest the elbow on a table with the small finger against your cheek. Then trace the color along the roots from the outside corners to the inside.

1. Upper lids. Look down and gently draw the pen/pencil along the roots of the lashes but not too close to the inner corners, where color collects. For evening, make the line wider over the pupil of the eye as you look straight into the mirror. Taper the line as it reaches the outer corner. This makes the eyes appear larger.

2. Lower lids. Look up and draw color along the roots of the lower lashes from outer to inner corners, leaving a small space open at the corners. Lining the entire lower lash line "closes" in the eye.

3. If you prefer, line only the outer two-thirds of the upper and/or lower lid.

Lining around the outer eye corners gives a theatrical look and tends to make eyes look smaller. If you like this, be sure it is not too dramatic for your face.

Adding Dimension to Special Eye Shapes _____

Close-set Eyes. (Eyes are close to the bridge of the nose). Place lightest shade of eye shadow on the inside area and darker shades on the outer area sweeping color up toward outer brow points. Start brow color further from the nose than the

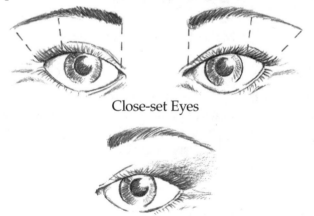

Close-set Eyes

Makeup for Close-set Eyes

Illustration 8

inner eye corner. Color the arch of your brow just beyond the outer edge of the iris. End the outer points of the brow slightly beyond the outer corner of eye. Line along the outer two-thirds and extend beyond the outer corners. Use lash-thickening mascara (see Illustration 8).

Wide-set Eyes. (Eyes are located further from the nose.) Place a shadow, foundation or concealer slightly darker than the skin tone on the inside areas of the eyes and down the side

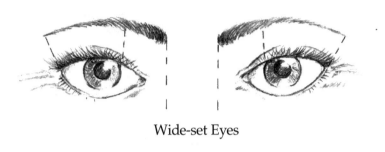

Wide-set Eyes

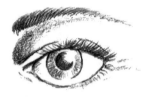

Makeup for Wide-set Eyes

Illustration 9

of the nose. Place a deeper shade in the crease of the eye and lighter one on the outer part. Start brow color closer to the nose than the inside corner and end it above the outer corner. The arch starts in front of the iris. Begin eye lining close to the inner corner and stop before reaching the outer corner (see Illustration 9).

Protruding Eyes. Blend a smoky to dark matte shadow from the upper lash line to the crease and slightly beyond the outer corners of the eyes, unless they are wide-set. Do not use white or anything pearlized on the lid. Use a medium shade from crease to brow with the lightest tone directly under the brow. A darker brow color "recedes" the protruding lids. Line both the upper and lower lids, smudging for softness. Emphasize the center of the eye with thicker mascara on the middle lashes (see Illustration 10).

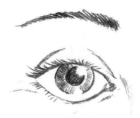
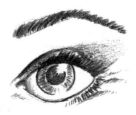

Illustration 10
Makeup for Protruding Eyes

Deep-set Eyes. Keep the eyebrow high and arched to give the illusion of more space. Place a light color—ivory or beige—on the lid from the lash line to the crease. Use a muted color like taupe or a soft brown, or one that matches clothing, above the crease and fan to outer brow. This is a triangle of color from the center of lid to outer brow point to the outer corner of the eye. Line outer one-half of lower lids and apply mascara (see Illustration 11).

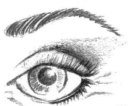

Illustration 11
Makeup for Deep-set Eyes

Small Eyes. Blend an ivory or soft taupe eye shadow on upper lids. Use a darker shade from crease up. Darker color on upper areas between crease and brow makes eyes appear larger, giving an upward focus.

Or, wrap color around
the outside corners.
See illustration 12a.

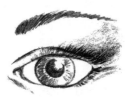

Illustration 12a

Or, form a dome over the center of each lid by applying a medium-to-dark shade from lash line to slightly above crease. Use a pale shade directly under brows.

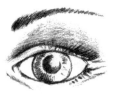

Illustration 12b

Do not use dark shades to line. They "shut in" the eyes. Line the entire upper lid, and rim the lower one from the center to slightly beyond the outer corner. Blue eyeliner along the lower lashes accentuates the whites of the eyes and makes them appear larger. Use lash-thickening mascara.

Drooping Upper Lids. Use a pale eye shadow on lids from the lash line to the crease. Place a darker shadow from the lash line to outer brow points, covering the droop. Apply mascara to outer one-half of upper and lower lashes and thicker mascara on the lashes in the center of upper lids. Begin lining from inner corner and taper off before reaching the outer corner (see Illustration 13).

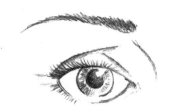 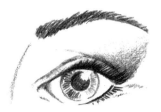

Illustration 13
Camouflaging Drooping
Upper Lids

Oriental or Asian. These eyes have minimal lids, which may appear to protrude or disappear. For shadow, try the earth tones—taupe, woody browns, olive, grey or charcoal. Blend a medium-toned shadow or foundation to the inner eye area to increase the contour from the inner eye to the inner brow corners. Use a darker shade from the lashes to midway between the lid and brow then fade out the color up towards the brow with the lightest shade directly under the brow. Brush mascara to the outer two-thirds of the lashes. Using an eye lining pen for a delicate trim, trace color along the base of the lashes (see Illustration 14).

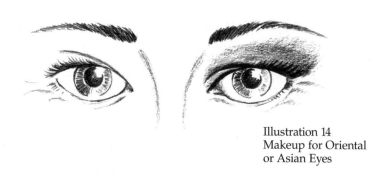

Illustration 14
Makeup for Oriental
or Asian Eyes

Cosmetic Tattooing. An innovation to adding facial color is permanent cosmetic tattooing of eyebrows, lining eyelids and lips. Softening scars and port wine stains with tattooing has been around a long time but only recently has cosmetic tattooing been refined as a substitute for loss of brows and lashes and even for drawing natural-looking nipples on women who have had mastectomies and want breast reconstruction.

The growing popularity of cosmetic tattooing equates with the increasing number of women past 50 who choose to remain active in work and play. For women whose brows and lashes are sparser or lighter and for busy women who are crunching time, it eliminates at least two steps in makeup application. Just think—you can wake up in the morning, get out of the pool, ski or hike, with forever-young brows and defined eyes.

Shapely brows and eye lining via cosmetic tattooing can easily erase years from the face. When done by an artistic expert, they look as natural as the originals and sometimes better. One woman who was 84 with failing eyesight wanted brows added and lids lined before she became blind.

Lips that are imperfect or have an indefinite outline can be made shapelier by cosmetic tattooing. Some women may not even need lipstick during daytime. Cheeks can be tattooed to add color but, generally, the result is less than perfect and may look unnatural.

A skilled cosmetic tattooist should have a good educational background in the field and related experience plus a keen sense of what colors are becoming to the client. Color can always be added so a conservative beginning is best. It's advisable to have a patch test to resolve questions about the right shade.

When cosmetic tattooing is done by a qualified technician in the United States, there is little possibility of infection. The skin is anesthetized topically and new sterilized needles are used every time pigment is implanted into the skin.

Since only a few states register cosmetic tattooists, you may need to call your State Board of Cosmetology or a board certified plastic surgeon. Not all states regulate cosmetic tattooing. "Do not go to a body tattooist listed in the classified section of the telephone book," advises Madelyn Stengel who is registered by the Colorado Board of Cosmetology and is also a teacher of cosmetic interdermal tattooing. She is recommended by hospitals, dermatologists and plastic surgeons. Her work involves adding color enhancement to the face, tattooing life-like nipples on reconstructed breasts, and diminishing the appearance of scars on the face and body.

She advises that when you find a cosmetic tattooist, ask for the names of three or four of their clients, talk to them, observe the work, or look at before-and-after photographs.

After you have talked to the tattooist, ask yourself: Do I like her? Does she understand what I want? Was she easy to talk to and did she take the time to deal with my concerns? Madelyn's advice is be wary, proceed with caution, get what you want—not what the tattooist wants, and have realistic expectations.

Cheeks

Cheer up your cheeks with color! If your choice is to wear very little makeup, blush is imperative. Faces seem lifeless without it. Blush or rouge enlivens the face with color that is naturally associated with health and well-being and gives sparkle to the eyes by showing off their jewel tones.

Too many women apply it in dabs instead of blends. Blush should appear realistic, like it comes from within. This happens when the complexion is properly primed, tinted with foundation, and the blush is seen as shimmering color.

Creme blush is usually preferred for dry skin and powder blush for oily, but, you can use either one or both. Apply creme rouge, then dust with powder blush for longer-lasting color. Darker shades give more shape to the face than the lighter ones.

Placement. Identify the triangle from the top of your ears to the lower edge of the nose to the bottom tip of the ears. Bring the color to the middle of the ear. This is the general area for placement. Now, look straight into the mirror and find the point on the cheekbone directly below the pupil (see Illustration 15 on page 72). Blush does not go closer to the nose than this point, unless your face is wide. If this is the case, extend the blush closer to the nose.

Another way to find the proper placement is to use the cheekbone as a guide. Place three dots of color on the cheekbone—at the temple, below the outer edge of your brow and below the center of your eye. Blend toward the middle of the ears. If placed too close to the eye area above the cheekbone, it detracts from the iris and draws attention to puffiness and crow's feet.

The Long Face. Keep the blush on the cheekbone to break the vertical line. Blend blush across the lower chin area.

The Wide Face. Take the color slightly closer to the nose and down to the jawbone at the sides of the face.

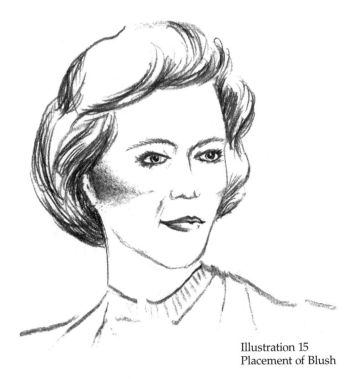

Illustration 15
Placement of Blush

Fleshy Cheeks. To get more contour, place a darker shade of blush under the cheekbone, starting below the outside corners of the eyes and drawing it toward the ears. As with all contouring, blend the edges to be sure the effect, not the technique, is apparent.

Pointed Chin. Soften by blending blush under the chin.

Cheekbones. Blush placed high on the cheekbones emphasizes them and accentuates the shadows beneath.

Eyeglasses. Blush should glow around the outside corners of the frames.

Do Something Different with Blush.

1. From the point on the cheekbone below the pupil, brush color up to and around the temples, as far over as the

middle of the brows forming a parenthesis of color to frame the eyes. Blend the edges.

2. For the sun-kissed look, sweep it across cheeks and down the nose.

3. If you have a high exposed forehead, tint the center just below the hairline.

Lips

Lip color perks up the whole face with a variety of hues from clear salmon pinks to deep plums, from lush wines to intense berries. Good lip products combat dryness and moisturize.

Lip Lining. Miracles are achieved with makeup especially when it comes to lips. Perfectly shaped lips are rare, but they materialize when properly outlined. Notice the pictures in fashion magazines and see how their lips have been enlarged to a fuller shape. You can do it, too.

One woman in a makeup class said she had a stroke, and the left side of her upper lip was lower than the right side. I showed her how to line the low side slightly higher to match the right side. The correction was easy, and her lips now had equal proportions (see Illustration 16).

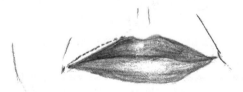

Illustration 16
Lip Lining to Perfect Shape

To shape lovely lips the pencil lip liner and sharpener are indispensable. If the point continues to break, return the product and get an automatic lip liner. One liner in a warm or cool shade can work for all your lipsticks because lip color is blended into the line with a lip blush. When the color is not brushed into the line, the result is unnatural and hard-looking.

For small lips trace a thin line outside the natural lip border.

When the borders are uneven, draw them even.

If one lip is small and the other large, line the small portion outside the border and the larger, inside.

A round face has better proportion with sharply defined lips.

A narrow face is softened by fuller, rounder lips.

If the outer corners droop, uptilt the corners with a wider line above the upper lip corners.

Color. Light, bright shades make small lips look larger. Dark or muted colors make large lips look smaller. Rich reds or sunny pink-corals de-emphasize the double chin. Some faces look dull without a bright lip color. This is because the undertones of the skin demand vivid shades. Also, if clothing has vibrant tones, the makeup should reflect this. Dark clothing colors and evening wear call for a deeper or brighter lip color.

Mixing colors increases your palette. Maybe that color you're not crazy about will be great when combined with another one.

You "soften" the lines surrounding the lips by using a color with a matte, non-shiny finish.

> When the bow shape of the upper lip is pronounced, it gives unnecessary sharpness to the mouth. Soften by drawing a line across the lower part of the dip. Fill in with lipstick.
>
>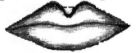

Tips for Application and Longer-Lasting Color.

1. Apply a creme foundation around the lip border, stretching them across the teeth to get the product into the fine lines. This disguises the lines and covers broken capillaries. Foundation placed on the inside of the lips may cake.

2. Outline as described and press translucent powder on this area.

3. Fill in with a lip brush rather than the lipstick itself. This gives a thinner coat which lasts longer than a thick coat. Use a light color on a thin upper lip (to make it appear fuller) and a darker shade on a full lower lip (to make it thinner) or vice versa for symmetry. Blot, until no color comes off.

4. Lipstick brands with a stain or fewer emollients stay on better.

Feathering.

When lip color seeps into the fine lines around the mouth and looks smeared, it is called feathering or bleeding. The gradual loss of collagen in this area causes a blurring of the border between the lip and the skin. But, don't despair. Here are some ways to restrain wandering color:

1. Moisturizers with collagen temporarily plump up the lines.

2. Apply a lip conditioner or primer before your color.

3. Be sure to get your foundation in the lines around the lips. Creme or powder creme foundation fills in the lines better than liquid foundation.

4. Outlining the lips holds the color in.

5. Some lipsticks are advertised as non-bleeding.

6. A dermatologist can inject collagen into the lines, plumping up and redefining the lip border. The procedure also adds lost volume to thinning lips. Touch-ups are required every six months or so.

Flaky Lips. Dab petroleum jelly onto moist lips. Gently slough away flakes with a soft tooth brush or dry terry washcloth. An alpha hydroxy acid product may also help this condition.

Black, Hispanic and Asian Skin

Cosmetic colorings bestow an exotic glamour on these complexions. If you have never played up your color with flattering makeup, now is the time. Ayo Vaughan Richards' book *Black and Beautiful* graphically describes the why's and how's to realizing beauty potential for darker skin tones.

Skin Care. Use non-irritating products, alcohol/fragrance free and oil-free if skin is oily. Exfoliation and masking are important. Moisturize dry areas, especially around the eyes where wrinkles are most likely to appear first. All skin types including darker tones need sun protection whenever necessary; use a non-sensitizing product.

Foundation. Use one that is water-based and oil-free. The shade that blends skin tones and brightens eyes is the right one.

Cheeks/Lips. Warm or cool skin tones determine your best color choices. Some suggestions are: For the lighter skin— coral, mauve, red, amber; for medium-tones—rose, brick, copper, russet; for ebony—wine, bronze, burgundy, dark red. To tone down red, mix with tinted lip gloss or foundation.

To make full lips smaller, line the lips inside the normal lip border with a raisin or burgundy lip liner. Fill in with a dark shade of lipstick.

Eyes. Ayo Vaughan-Richards calls them the windows of your soul, the mirror of your personality and a reflection of your beauty.[6] Eyes with added color are more expressive. Behind glasses, use heavier liner, shadow and mascara.

Shadow. For black brown irises use black, dark brown,

navy blue, dark green, purple, rust, or mauve. For other eye colors see the previous section on Eye Shadow, **Guidelines for Selecting Eye Shadow Colors,** page 61. When a color is too bright, tone it down with brown or beige.

Shadow Highlighters. Depending upon your skin tone, use golden-bronze, beige, pale mauve, violet, dusty pink. Add glamour to evening wear with the metallic glint of gold-bronze or copper in the temple area, the outer corner of the brows, or the outside corner of your cheekbone. Carefully fade out the glitter.

Liners. If black is too harsh, use grey or brown. For more color use dark blue, wine or purple, especially if they imitate clothing colors.

Translucent Powder. Select the shade that goes with your skin. Powdering gives a matte finish and absorbs excess oil. When oil reappears, pat dry with blotting papers and dust again.

Makeovers

All women are over 50. The photos are not retouched to conceal lines or wrinkles. As in Magic of Makeup classes, the women applied their own makeup with my guidance. For all three, I added brow color above the inner points to restore the youthful lift. In the "after" pictures, all wear a quality foundation that gives good coverage.

> With care, color and know-how, we can take age out of image.

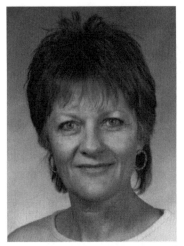
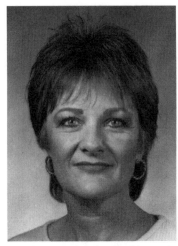

Judy—medical recruiter. Her foundation even conceals freckles. We enriched her eyes with brow color and black lash-thickening mascara. She always lines her eyes ... calls it her "trademark." Lining the eyes makes the whites whiter. Eye shadow is shades of brown. We drew lips fuller with a lip definer pencil and filled in with a rich red.

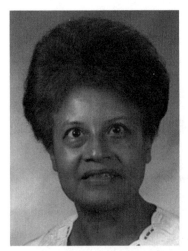
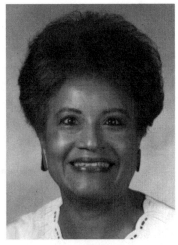

Patricia—administration coordinator. We used an ivory concealant to lighten eye areas, extended and darkened the brows with black brow pencil, then used black mascara and shadow with black eye liner. Blush was blended from the upper ear tip to mid-ear and lower ear tip to directly below the pupils on the cheek bone. Her smile adds sparkle to her eyes.

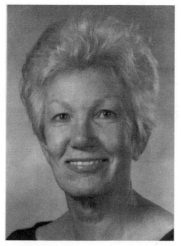 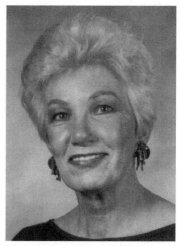

Margaret—owner of an insurance agency. Ruddiness was toned down with a concealant before applying foundation. We added width and color to brows with a taupe brow pencil and eye shadow in tones of brown diminishing darker shade to above the brow bone. She has full lips with deep color and gets the best shade by using an underbase before she applies a medium shade of lip color. Unlike Judy and Patricia, blush is shaped parallel with check bones to balance facial length—not triangular as described for Patricia.

The Professional Finish

Translucent powder is fine textured and available in different shades. It can be pressed as in compacts or loose. Pressed powder is tops for touchups and zapping T-zone (mid-forehead, nose area and chin) shine. Keep loose powder for home use. This sheer powder offsets the facial shine of some moisturizing foundations that tend to exaggerate lines. It also helps makeup to last longer and softens the colors. If it dulls any of your colorings, especially the blush, you have applied too much.

Sparingly, dust the facial hairs down. If powder collects in the lines, it emphasizes them. If your skin is dry, even a light dusting with translucent powder may settle in the lines or accentuate a flaky texture. Some powders actually draw oil and moisture from the skin.

Women with dry skin may prefer to mist their face by using a commercial spray such as Evian, or make your own. Put mineral water (tap water may have too many chemicals) into a small atomizer with a very fine spray. Add the liquid from one vitamin E capsule and a couple drops of perfume oil. This atomizer is easily carried in your purse. Besides adding a dewy get-up and glow, it "sets" the makeup for dry skin the way powder does for combination/oily skin.

> The extra time spent to apply foundation carefully is the base for a natural, professional finish.

For the working woman, a mid-day spritz hydrates thirsty skin and won't muss makeup. The small atomizer is also handy for women who travel and experience dehydration.

A Summary on Using Makeup for Face Lifts ———

Inner Brows. If the inner points of your brows curve downward, add brow color above these points to balance with the middle of the brows.

Eyes. Lighten shadowy areas around eyes, especially the inner corners. Give your eyes a lift by slanting shadow upward, as in Illustration 6, blending well.

Coloration Around the Nose and Mouth. Ruddiness around the smile lines tends to "drag down" the face. Lighten these areas with a concealer or foundation.

"Lifting the Lines." Using a very pale concealer or foundation, blend from the outside corners of the eyes and/or brows up toward the hairline. Fade out edges into the tinting foundation. The width of this shading depends upon the width of the temple.

Diminishing the Lines. Using a thin, pointed brush, or a sponge tip, place pale or white concealant or foundation in the bottom of the line. Pat gently, being careful not to blend it off. Dust with powder and cover with tinting foundation.

The Double Chin. With foundation or a concealant one or two shades darker than your regular one, start at the bottom center of your chin and blend to the right and left then slightly under the chin but not down the throat—a triangle of shading. Blend. A classic red lip color draws attention away from a double chin (see Illustration 17).

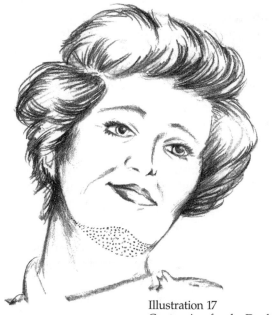

Illustration 17
Contouring for the Double Chin

Eyeglasses

Makeup. Makeup increases the significance of eyes especially when they are behind glasses. Since tinted lenses darken the eye area, you can add definition by lining the upper and lower lids and lighten with eye shadow. A generous application of mascara adds more definition. If eye makeup is not an option, give extra care to lipstick and blush so that it is not covered by the frames.

If you are farsighted, the lenses of your glasses make your eyes appear larger. Wear eye shadow in subdued shades. If you are nearsighted, the lenses make eyes look smaller; use bolder colors.

Frames. Since people often see the glasses before the eyes, shop for the best fitting frames that complement all your features and hair. Insist that they don't slip down but rest on the nose not on the cheeks. The pupils of the eyes need to be as close to the center of the lenses as possible.

Upward tilting frames or high temples provide a lift at the sides of the face. Elongated frames, wide from temple to temple, give the face a droopy-eyed look. For crow's feet, opt for side pieces hooked to the bottom of the lenses. A low bridge interrupts the vertical line of a long nose and rimless frames tend to make the face look older.

Guidelines for Selecting Frames.

If your face is:	Frames should be:
Oval	Squarish, usually any style but extremes; with a very thin oval use frames for the oblong/rectangle shape.
Square	Curved or oval.
Wide	No wider than outer corners of the eyes and longer from brows to cheeks than they are wide from nose to temples.
Oblong/Rectangle	Angular to shorten the long face and wider from nose to temples than they are from brows to cheeks.
Round	Angular or hexagonal, not round.
Inverted Triangle	Round or square.
Fair-skinned	Lightweight metals or plastic in crystal, light beige, rose, lavender.
Dark-skinned	Bright metal colors like white gold, pink lilac, raspberry, emerald.

Sunglasses. According to the American Academy of Ophthalmology,[7] studies reveal that large amounts of visible blue and violet and invisible ultraviolet light that are found in the sun's rays can be harmful to the eyes. These rays accelerate the aging and deterioration of human vision and play a major role in the formation of cataracts.

Consequently, sunglasses have a definite healthful purpose besides being a glamorous fashion accessory. It is advisable to wear them year-round to safeguard the sensitive thin skin around the eye area and to prevent squint lines.

To avoid color distortion and still have good screening from the ultraviolet A and B (UVA and UVB) rays, lenses in dark grey, green or a combination with brown have proven to be satisfactory. Lenses tinted pink, purple, and especially blue distort color perception (for example: traffic lights) and are usually not dark enough for effective blocking. Look for the words "special purpose" or "blocks 99 percent of ultraviolet (UV) rays." Some block 100 percent. "Cosmetic" or "fashion" sunglasses block 70 percent or less.

Wraparound sunglasses prevent the ultraviolet rays from sneaking past the top, bottom and sides. The best are snug fitting or curved to fit the face, with opaque or ultraviolet blocking side shields.

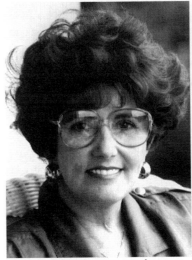
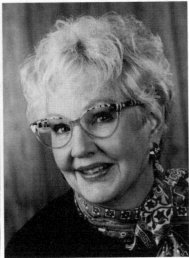

Frames courtesy of
Optical Sales, Portland, OR

Frames courtesy of
Europtics, Inc. Denver, CO

Your face deserves a flattering frame.

Excess Facial Hair

Any time after 40 women grow more facial hair and sometimes a few coarse ones because of changes in the hormonal balance.

During a makeup class one woman exclaimed, "Just look at all the hair on my face! I'm so embarrassed by it. It's terrible!" She was surprised to find out that no one else had noticed this "terrible" hair. People view us from at least three feet away and seldom see the things that make us self-conscious.

Tweezing is recommended for the few, coarse hairs. Warm wax removal of superfluous hair is easy and quick. The only discomfort is a momentary smarting when the wax is pulled off. With this process the hair grows back fine and soft without a stubble. Regrowth takes four to six weeks.

This is a job for the professional, not the amateur, because the wax has to be the right temperature, and the skin must be held a certain way when removing the wax. Many salons as well as beauty schools offer this service. The cost at beauty schools is reasonable and some have senior discounts.

After several professional treatments, you may feel you know the procedure well enough to try a cold wax removal and do it yourself. A chemical or wax depilatory removes the hair at the surface, and within a few days stubbles can be seen and felt. To avoid stubbles, find a product that removes the hair by the roots and follow the manufacturer's instructions.

Stay Up-to-Date!!

How many times have we wished we had someone's opinion on new ideas we want to try? If you have one or two good friends and you like the way they do their faces, get together and experiment with different techniques or colors. Maybe they want advice, too. Take advantage of every opportunity to learn about makeup.

Pictures in women's magazines illustrate the current modes of facial design. Even if the models are young, we can observe the trends and adapt them to fit our style. The *Town and Country* magazine has beautiful photos of stylish women who are over 40. Browsing through fashion magazines, you find out what's current and what's worth buying in the market of multi-faceted cosmetic products. Occasionally, there are articles about makeovers, surveys of new products, and advice from experts on hair, makeup, and skin care as well as information from models and celebrities about what works for them.

Makeup for the Occasion

The occasion and the time of day influence how and what makeup we should wear. Keep the face attractive and timeless whether the occasion is casual or formal.

When participating in exercise classes, athletics, hiking, etc., wear minimal makeup. I was on a group hike and one of the women wore eye makeup suitable for a cocktail party. By the end of the hike her shadow was spotty and eye liner, smearing. She really looked worn-out, and maybe she was, but the runaway makeup didn't help.

Minimal makeup still looks finished. For sheer base color, try one of the following:

- Your regular liquid foundation
- Equal parts of liquid foundation and a moisturizer
- A liquid foundation formulated with a moisturizer
- A moisturizer formulated with a tint
- A self-tanning oil, creme or lotion

Then add brow color, blush and a trace of lipstick. If you have good lip pigmentation, you may want only a touch of lip gloss. For small pale lips, rim them with lip liner and add color.

If you are going from an afternoon activity to an evening

engagement, deepen your daytime colors. To dramatize the eyes with shadow, sweep it subtly from the outer corners up toward the temples to give more lift. Maybe you want a wedge of shadow around the outer eye corners and/or a tinge of shading along the lower lashes. Touch up the eye lining. Give blush a dash more color and redo the lips. Set with either a dusting of powder or misting.

Night-time colorings are more daring and satiny than daytime. Makeup helpers such as Zero Base by Clinique or Blanc de Chanel, applied under your foundation, give the face a translucent finish. They brighten the dull or sallow complexion, even out skin tones, and fill in tiny lines. Use sparingly. Add a dot of gloss to the center of your lips and a pale shadow with sheen directly under the brow, not on lines or wrinkles.

––––––––––

Once you start working with different colorings, your imagination will be stimulated to be more creative. You'll catch yourself thinking, "I wonder how this would look ..." Go with that. Keep following your hunches, and you'll soon see how makeup reveals the winning image.

> Avoid being a fade-out. Promise yourself to touch-up makeup mid-day, mid-evening, mid-occasion, whenever necessary and convenient. Most makeup fades in two to three hours depending on the oiliness of the skin and the quality of the product.

4

You Can Brighten Your Smile

Two ways to brighten a smile are to straighten and whiten our teeth. Why straighten teeth after mid-life? A few of the reasons are:

- To maintain long-term health of teeth and gums,

- To keep the jaw line age-resistant,

- To feel the physical and psychological lift of an attractive, pleasing smile.

I did it way past mid-life and have never been sorry.

"Our faces and facial expressions are two of the truest reflections of the way we feel about ourselves." Tom Linnell, a psychologist practicing in Ft. Collins, Colorado said. "If we have to hide our faces in embarrassment, it means we're also hiding part of ourselves. Being able to smile openly brightens our whole personality."[2]

Many people past 40 are having their teeth straightened because of longstanding discomfort, teeth moving into peculiar positions, or they are just fed up with the embarrassment of crooked teeth. To hide imperfect alignment people adopt mannerisms or never smile. Today, men and women over 40, 50, even 60 and 70, are asking: Why not straighten those teeth that have bothered me all these years?

Orthodontia for this group has tripled in the last decade. Almost everyone I talked to knew someone age forty or more who had had their teeth straightened, or they themselves had the treatment. Amazingly few people are born with teeth in perfect alignment.

Once a boyfriend in high school said to me, "You wouldn't be bad-looking if that tooth didn't stick out." As the years rolled by my bite worsened, and after the second grandchild, I began to consider doing something about it. The thought of a steely smile kept putting me off, so I asked friends, "What do you think about my wearing braces?" As I wondered if they would think of me as a foolish grandmother, I was shocked when, without exception, the replies were, "Go for it!" They all knew at least one person over 40 who was happy with orthodontic correction.

In my quest for further confirmation, I talked with persons who had tested the waters. Betty, a supervisor and landsman with an oil company, said the year she turned 50 was depressing the whole twelve months. Facing increased competition from younger personnel and wanting a business career for 15 to 20 more years, she realized self-improvement was imperative.

First, she lost 15 pounds and whittled her figure into shape. Then, she had her upper teeth capped and at 55, the lower ones were straightened. Since her teen years, she had always been self-conscious about her mouth. One tooth actually sat sideways. This was corrected by wearing braces for six months and a retainer for a year.

She was amazed at how easily and efficiently the correction was made and wished she had done it years before "because it turned out to be such a simple thing." There is no question in her mind that a youthful, healthy appearance is important on the professional scene.

Ellie, a woman in her 70s, said her lower teeth were moving in such a way that they lacerated her lip. When she decided to have them straightened, her husband thought she was crazy and asked, "What's an old woman like you straightening her teeth for?" In eight months her teeth were even, and she had experienced no pain or discomfort with the braces. Only the habitual brushing three times a day was bothersome. If she hadn't done it, her lower teeth would still be cutting her lip. Not only did her teeth look a lot better, but her gums were healthier.

When I came back from the orthodontist's office with metallic contraptions on, I was surprised when someone said, "You look younger!" and another thought I looked cute"! Besides the association of braces with the very young, the brackets plumped out the lines around my lips. But my mouth felt cluttered, and I didn't want to smile that first week, let alone eat. My daughter advised me not to worry about smiling because it only attracted more attention to the braces, and "Besides," she said, "they're not that noticeable."

Most of the people who commented about them had either worn braces, knew people over 40 who had, or wished their teeth were straighter. It was exciting to see the teeth moving into line and realize that for the first time in my life I was going to have a smile that didn't have a tinge of self-consciousness.

Dr. Daryl R. Burns, D.D.S., has been practicing orthodontics for 28 years and his current patients include not only the young people but also many who are 40 to 80 years old. He said repositioning teeth in adulthood takes longer and is not as easy or efficient as it is in childhood. But, successful corrections are completed; the teeth do move.

Coequal to the advantage of straight teeth is the re-education in oral hygiene, an indispensable part of the orthodontic procedure. The American Dental Association contends that, with good oral hygiene, your teeth can last a lifetime.[3]

Besides the cosmetic advantage, straight teeth contribute to dental health. They are easier to clean, and there's less stress to the surrounding gum tissue. This means a reduction in the risk of teeth loosening, gum disease, and the loss of gum, bone, or teeth.

For the duration of the treatment, the patient must punctuate the day with brushings, flossing and the use of a Water Pik® or similar cleaning machine. Cleaning machines make the routine easier and better. The Water-Pik shoots a stream of water at different speeds, washing out particles between the teeth that are not probed by brushing. The force of the spray massages the gums and leaves a squeaky-clean mouth. Conscientious orthodontic clients probably have the cleanest mouths in town, and the pleasantness is likely to make the routine permanent.

To meet the requirements for orthodontic treatment, the patient must be highly motivated—willing to put time into the cleansing routine, because if the teeth and braces are not kept clean, gum tissues could become inflamed. And she must have healthy gums and bone. There is the risk of root resorption or of a tooth becoming non-vital from movement. These problems don't occur very often because periodic x-rays and frequent examinations of gum tissue help to prevent them. Present-day appliances with resilient wires, not rigid and tough as they used to be, also reduce risks. Pain is inconsequential in modern orthodontia.

The biggest bugaboo is vanity. Fortunately, the industry has come out with porcelain-type brackets that are clear with flesh-colored ties. Some of the self-consciousness of a metallic grin is removed with these new appliances. All this is a small inconvenience compared to the enduring advantages of a healthy bite and even teeth.

According to Dr. Burns, straight teeth and oral hygiene aren't the total answer to dental health. They must be combined with checkups and a diet that gives the teeth plenty of exercise through chewing fresh fruits and vegetables.

Dr. Burns said that straight teeth "build up one's self-confidence to have a smile that goes from ear to ear and to feel good about doing it. There are a lot of people walking around who do not smile because their teeth are irregular. When you converse with someone, it's a great feeling to know you have an even set of teeth."

Whitening. Dull, dingy teeth can be improved to a shiny, youthful white according to Donald L. Finks, D.D.S. of Denver, Colorado. Unsmiling women with embarrassing yellow teeth find new freedom of expression when teeth are whitened. It literally changes personalities. "A smile says much more than words," Dr. Finks said. "It expresses the warmth of an individual's personality and makes a remarkable difference." And, to women who associate with people on a career, service or social basis, a sparkling smile is a big bonus.

Stains are classified as two kinds: Extrinsic stains result from cigarettes, cigars, coffee, tea, red wine, and some medications. These are easier to remove than intrinsic stains. Intrinsic stains are incorporated in the enamel and will not lighten quite as well.

The process is simple and painless, consisting of wearing clear plastic guards or trays that are customized to fit the teeth and contain a bleaching gel. This is a 10% solution of carbamide peroxide which has been used for years as an oral antiseptic. The trays can be worn on either the uppers or lowers or both from bedtime to awakening. Eighty to 100 hours of soaking teeth in the bleaching gel is required, depending on the nature of the discoloration. Teeth can get up to four shades lighter after five to six nights of treatment, but there is no way to predict results.

One year after the initial whitening a touchup is advised for several days. If smoking and coffee are in the picture, restaining occurs quicker and touchups will be needed more often. The whitening process does not replace regular professional cleaning and daily oral hygiene.

Whitening is easier on the pocketbook than capping, bonding or veneers. Compared to these, it is a relatively inexpensive way to keep an attractive smile *at any age.* Cost normally ranges from $200 to $400.

This is just one of the many facets of the large and rapidly growing field of cosmetic dentistry. Most cities have a dental society with a referral service to identify doctors who do cosmetic dentistry.

Teeth aren't extracted now as often as they were in past decades. It's no longer a fact that dentures are in our future. Dr. Finks has patients in their 70s and 80s—one is 96—who still have their own teeth. This is the trend. "We can't improve on the Guy who made them," Dr. Finks emphasized. Compared to people who have their originals, denture wearers take three times as long to masticate their food. With regular dental hygiene and daily brushing, the expectancy is that the majority of people will keep their teeth for a lifetime, and they can be pearly white, too.

5

Erasing the Wrinkles

"I've never liked the way I looked
and you know what that does to
your self-esteem. [At 71] I've
never looked so good in my
entire life."
—Phyllis Diller[1] (after many
facial and dental corrections)

The continual evolution of ideas on good mental and physical health habits increases the possibility of a one-hundred-year lifespan, filled with multiple occupations, careers and service oriented jobs. Nowadays many women have two vocations—one as homemaker and a job, sometimes two, outside the home. It's not unusual for women to spend ten to twenty years in one occupation, and then re-educate themselves for entirely different work.

Longevity is acceptable if health, useful activity and appearance inspire a sense of self-worth. The double standard of aging—wrinkles on men are okay but not on women—is just one reason why women want to erase them. Dr. Maxwell Maltz, a plastic surgeon, says many need a better self-image. This alone is sufficient justification. If eliminating a few lines and wrinkles or other unsightly skin problems relieves chronic unhappiness (a very real malady), the money is well spent.[2]

Dale Alexander[3] reiterates Dr. Maltz's statement when he says that overhauling the skin can prove to be very gratifying.

It's a far healthier response than withdrawing into a depressive state. But, if we don't nourish the skin with healthy habits, unattractive textures gradually reappear. Beneficial eating, daily exercise, complexion care, and correct makeup application should be established as a daily routine. A surgeon said that frequently women who have had cosmetic surgery don't know how to further enhance it with makeup.

There are many ways to erase the wrinkles. Here are a few.

Retin-A

Retin-A, a derivative of vitamin A acid, is a prescriptive drug, patented and manufactured by Ortho Pharmaceutical Corporation, a division of Johnson & Johnson. It is a topical treatment available in a gel, cream or liquid, to be used under the supervision of a dermatologist. At first, application may cause some discomfort. Research is continuing in order to find a retinoid that does not cause redness, dryness or peeling.

In her book *How to be Wrinkle-Free,* Carlotta Karlson Jacobson, Beauty Editor of *Harper's Bazaar*[4] comments favorably on Retin-A because she uses it and has received many compliments on her lovely complexion. Retin-A diminishes fine wrinkles, resulting in a smoother texture, but it does not improve deep furrows or sagging skin. Lines may reappear if treatment is discontinued.

Skin medicated with Retin-A is super sensitive to climatic changes and sun rays. Applying the product in the evening, thoroughly rinsing it off in the morning and using a fragrance-free sun block with an SPF of 15 or more gives the needed protection. Since the process is drying, moisturizing is very important. If there is a reaction, application should be discontinued, and your doctor advised.

Collagen Injections _____

Collagen is a natural protein found throughout the body. It provides the skin with structural support, form and resiliency. Wrinkles and sagging occur when the collagen decreases during the aging process causing facial depressions.

Collagen in moisturizers works on the skin's surface as a temporary cap to help the skin retain water.

Collagen injections are made of highly purified bovine collagen that is similar to human collagen and readily accepted by the body. It is injected into the skin to supplement the body's own collagen. Injections fill in lines and furrows such as those on the forehead and around the eyes, nose and mouth. Scars are minimal, and the texture of the skin is improved.

Relatively painless and costing less than major cosmetic surgery, the collagen injection procedure involves:

1. A skin test. There is a small risk of allergic reaction. About three percent of those tested have negative reactions.

2. A series of treatments. Injections are directed below the surface of the skin where contour problems begin. Injectable collagen treatments are not meant for people who have excess facial skin or for those who want a major resurfacing of the skin.

3. Periodic touch-ups. One treatment is not permanent. Follow-up injections require less collagen than the first treatment. They are necessary to maintain maximum correction and may be needed every six to twelve months. The length of time between treatments depends upon the patient's skin and reaction to the collagen.

Pamphlets on collagen injection are available from Customer Relations, Collagen Corporation, 2500 Faber Place, Palo Alto, CA 94303. This information answers some of the most frequently asked questions, but does not take the place of a consultation with a qualified physician.

*Acid Chemical Peels*_____

This procedure has been around for about fifty years. It is a low-risk regenerative procedure that erases lines, tightens facial wrinkles without surgery, and makes dull skin look radiant. Wrinkles around the mouth and eyes respond well, but this process is not effective for hanging skin folds.

Individuals with fair complexions respond better than those with darker skin. It is not recommended for people with kidney, liver and lung problems.

In most cases, one treatment is enough. Results have been known to last as long as 20 years. If the wrinkling was due to sun exposure and/or alcohol and tobacco, and the individual continues exposure to these elements, wrinkles will return. Peels are very effective in treating sun-damaged skin. The bleaching effect can also remove dark under-eye circles. Chemical peels rejuvenate the skin by burning off the top layers with acid compounds, erasing age spots, wrinkles, sallowness and blotchiness that have accumulated on the top layer of the skin and leaving a clearer, younger-looking complexion. Some experts believe that penetration to the underlying dermis also stimulates a fresh new growth of natural collagen.

The procedure takes one to one and one-half hours to apply the chemical to the skin. After four to six days a crust is removed revealing a smoother, softer, and firmer textured skin beneath. After about eight days in the hospital, the patient goes home. Follow-up visits are continued for a year to monitor the progress.

A light chemical peel only takes about twenty minutes with a healing period of three to five days.

Dermabrasion _____

Dermabrasion works best with firm parts of the face, such as the forehead and the nose, while the chemical peel is especially suited for areas where the skin isn't rigid such as around the lips. Some physicians combine dermabrasion and the chemical peel, using a mechanical resurfacer for deep wrinkles and acid for large areas of lighter wrinkles.

Both peels and dermabrasions leave the face raw-looking for 10 to 14 days until the new layer of skin appears. The most serious problem with dermabrasion is that the new skin is lighter in color than the unabraded skin. This is not as much of a problem for pale complexions as it is for darker skin. Because of the lighter pigmentation of the new skin, doctors have found it necessary to treat the whole face rather than specific areas.

Surgery _____

Rhytidectomy (surgical face-lifting), dermabrasion (rubbing away skin aberrations), skin peeling (acid applications) and collagen injections are used in plastic surgery. The word plastic is derived from the Greek word "plastikos," meaning molding or giving form.

To have or not to have a surgical facelift is a question that needs to be evaluated over a period of time, carefully considering the risks as well as the benefits and talking to women who have had one. Definite improvement is possible but women who expect perfection are often disappointed. If surgery is the choice, it is crucial to obtain a qualified and capable plastic surgeon by:

- Consulting your family physician or internist
- Calling the local County Medical Society
- Asking the local teaching or first class community hospital
- Writing the Executive Office of the American Society of Plastic and Reconstructive Surgeons, Inc., 444 E. Algonquin Road, Arlington Heights, IL 60005, or phone (800) 635-0635, the Patient Referral Service.

Be wary of exaggerated and sensational claims in the news media about plastic surgery or so-called "cosmetic surgeons" who are not board certified and whose training is not as comprehensive. They use a hard sell approach and may brush aside as inconsequential your concerns about safety.

Physicians who are certified by the American Board of Plastic Surgery must pursue post-graduate training of five to seven years that includes thorough grounding in general surgery and a minimum of two to three years in an approved plastic surgery training center. In addition, they are required to pass a rigorous examination in order to be officially certified by the American Board of Plastic Surgery or its Canadian equivalents, the Royal College of Physicians and Surgeons of Canada or the Corporation Professionelle du Medicin de Quebec.

The American Board of Plastic Surgery is the only board approved by the American Board of Medical Specialties for determining qualifications and certification in plastic surgery.

The certification of a physician by the American Board of Plastic Surgery does not guarantee perfect results. Medicine is an inexact art and postoperative results are dependent upon several contributing factors, which are sometimes unpredictable. But, the more thorough the surgeon's training, skill and experience, the greater the possibility for satisfactory results.

Responsible, ethical doctors should not mind answering these questions:

- Where do you have hospital privileges? Generally, this assures that the doctor has been reviewed by his or her peers.

- How safe is this operation?

- What are the potential side effects of the surgical procedure and how long will they last? Patients should know the side effects to determine when they will be able to resume normal activities.

- How much will this cost?

- How many of your patients have needed additional surgery to correct problems occurring from the original operation? The patient needs to know the probability of more surgical correction and if there will be an additional charge.

- May I contact former patients who have had the same surgical procedure that I want?

- What should I expect before, during, and after the operation?

If the doctor is unwilling to answer all of your concerns, find one who will.[5]

Betty Reed, 68, is an elegant five foot seven fashion model who began working as a television weather reporter over 30 years ago in Denver, Colorado. From there she went on to fashion modeling and has been active ever since in a career she loves. At 55 she realized she would be forced to stop working unless she did something about her wrinkling face. Her gynecologist recommended a plastic surgeon who was certified by the American Board of Plastic Surgery.

During the consultation she said she wanted to look like "the mother of the bride but a younger mother" in order to continue working. He explained exactly what had to be done and the risks. Since her health was good and her enthusiasm and determination high, she was a good candidate. The surgery took five hours and the results were very pleasing.

Although healing can take as long as six months, Betty heals fast. Two weeks after surgery she was on a modeling assignment in Colorado Springs. The only evidence was a little puffiness around the eyes, which soon disappeared. Silver haired, with a bubbly, sophisticated personality, she is the oldest, working runway model in Denver and enjoys every minute of it. She even edged out younger competition to land an assignment in the Bahamas.

Obviously, she is an advocate for cosmetic surgery. To her the biggest advantage was to be able to continue her modeling career, and the greatest improvement was to the eye area. Betty believes the risks are lessened if you have a competent doctor, but when you are on the operating table for five hours, risk is always present.

To maintain the health of her complexion she regularly follows a skin care regimen that "pays off" and takes plenty of vitamins A, C, E and kelp.

Her advice is to be very selective when choosing a doctor, and to "go for it when you are mentally prepared." Psychological preparation is crucial, and Betty was definitely psyched up. Do it for yourself, not for your husband or anyone else. Feeling good about your appearance ensures more self-confidence as well as the perks resulting from heightened self-esteem. "I felt better about me." Betty said. "It may not get a husband or a dream job, but there will be more possibilities."

A successful facelift is the result of: a well-prepared patient with the correct motivation and realistic expectations; anatomical characteristics of skin that are favorably conducive to surgery; and an expertly executed technical procedure.

Dr. George M. Lacy of Denver, Colorado, certified by the American Board of Surgery in 1965 and the American Board of Plastic Surgery in 1968, said that during a consultation the patient's motivation, actual physical condition, and medical history are discussed. He then explains the appropriate corrective procedure, pragmatic expectations and potential risks. If a client has unresolved neurotic or psychotic problems, or medical complications, it is not uncommon for a doctor to refuse to perform surgery even though the client believes she would benefit.

"The psychological element involved in evaluating the patient for cosmetic surgery is important both before and after surgery... We don't get involved in psycho therapy but the way a patient looks at herself both before and after surgery is very important," Dr. Lacy said.

If a woman between 60 and 65 is depressed because she looks haggard and tired but she doesn't feel it, and she wants to reenter the job market or have more social life, that woman is a good candidate.

In any type of surgery there are statistical risks such as bleeding, infection, unusual scar formation, and poor wound healing. This can happen even when the operation is properly done by a well-trained surgeon in a correct environment on a qualifiable patient. There are also complications unique to the procedures in the field of plastic surgery, but Dr. Lacy emphasized, usually everything works out fine, and the patient is pleased with the results.

Incisions are placed in a position where the hairline scars are inconspicuous and do not detract from the result. This may not always be the case, and during the consultation the client is forewarned.

In Dr. Lacy's opinion, "The three most harmful things that affect the skin over the years are overexposure to the sun, smoking and any overindulgence." Harmful exposure to the sun and smoking are the worst. Persons who tan heavily destroy a lot of the elastic fibers in the face, and they are more likely to have crinkly parchment-like skin as they age.

"We know that patients who smoke don't do as well with a facelift, or any kind of surgery, particularly skin flap surgery. A facelift does involve large skin flaps. In the smoker, the blood supply to the skin and face is significantly decreased, and the incidence of impaired circulation resulting in crusting, death of skin in the skin flaps, and excessive scarring is higher. This has become such a well-known fact that most plastic surgeons won't necessarily refuse to do a smoker, but almost all insist that the patient quits smoking at least one week before and one week after the operation."

Changes created by cosmetic surgery are subtle. The typical response from friends isn't, "Oh, you've had cosmetic surgery!" but "You look good, have you had a vacation?" or

"You must have slept well last night." After successful surgery the patient looks and feels better about herself. Usually, she has only one facelift and maybe periodic tucks. The amount of recurrent relifting differs with each client and depends upon the quality of the patient's skin, the shape of her face, the amount of fat under the skin, and the type of initial surgery.

It is important to protect the new complexion by conscientiously following the doctor's skin care advice especially for the first six to ten weeks and actually ever after. This includes a gentle water soluble cleanser, a moisturizer and an SPF 15 sunscreen. Women see the full afterglow of their investment when they learn how to wear makeup.

Whatever the remedy, find the best qualified and reputable dermatologist or surgeon to give you guidance and supervision.

On-going scientific research is continually improving upon the present procedures. Eventually the line-free complexion may be as easy as taking a pill and painless and safe for the majority of women.

The "Spiritual Facelift"

If a medical procedure is not desirable, ponder the suggestion of Dr. Maxwell Maltz, one of the world's most famous plastic surgeons, who practiced in England, Europe and South America:

"Try giving yourself a 'Spiritual Face Lift.' It is more than a play on words. It opens you up to more life, more vitality, the 'stuff' that youth is made of. You'll feel younger. You'll actually look younger. Many times I have seen a man or woman apparently grow five or ten years younger in appearance after removing old emotional scars. Look around you. Who are the youthful-looking people you know over the age of forty? The grumpy? Resentful? The pessimistic? The ones who are 'soured on the world,' or the cheerful, optimistic, good-natured people?

"Carrying a grudge against someone or against life can bring on the old age stoop, just as much as carrying a heavy weight around on your shoulders would. People with emotional scars, grudges, and the like are living in the past, which is characteristic of old people. The youthful attitude and youthful spirit erases wrinkles from the soul and the face,... looks to the future and has a great expectation...

"So why not give yourself a face lift? Your do-it-yourself kit consists of relaxation of negative tensions to prevent scars, ... creative living, a willingness to be a little vulnerable, and a nostalgia for the future instead of the past."*6

If you need further tools for this regenerative do-it-yourself kit, his book is loaded with them. Living need not be a waiting game. It can be attractive, active, useful and fulfilling.

---

* *Psycho-Cybernetics*, reprinted by permission of the publisher, Prentice Hall, a division of Simon & Schuster, Englewood Cliffs, NJ.

6

Hair

"Hair, like makeup, can be an
effective line hider."[1]
—Carlotta Karlson Jacobson

Unless you are wearing wild clothing colors or a spiked hairdo, the face assumes the focal point of your appearance with the hair complementing and adorning it. The hair should not compete with, overpower or detract from the face. It frames the face just as the brows frame the eyes.

Since regular exercise is good for the body, it is good for the hair, too. Bodily activity and massage bolster circulation. They also alleviate tensions, which can be harmful to the hair.

Proper maintenance is increasingly important as the hair begins to lose elasticity, moisture and volume. Hair is not self-sustaining. It needs consistent care and conditioning with products fortified with beneficial additives that strengthen and protect. These simple one-minute routines also help:

1. *Brushing.* The hair bordering the forehead and temples is more fragile. Brush this area with a gentle touch. Using a brush with wide-spaced bristles, bend over (either standing or sitting) and brush the hair down toward the floor, stroking from the nape of the neck to the forehead. Feel the bristles grazing the scalp where the life of the hair is. This stimulates the oil glands and increases the circulation. Do not overbrush. More than 15 strokes may be too much, especially for hair that breaks easily. Use your fingers to comb through, stroking the scalp with your nails.

2. *Massage.* A tight scalp may indicate poor circulation. To loosen, spread fingers firmly on your head and move the skin over the bone with the finger pads. Massage one area until it tingles then move on to the next. Enjoy the sensation of the blood flowing through the veins carrying its vital nutrients to the roots of the hair.

Nutrients. Hair is made from protein and thrives on it. Protein in the following foods strengthen and promote growth: fish, veal, eggs, chicken, turkey, beans, nuts, seeds, lowfat milk and cheese, fruits, vegetables (dark leafy greens like broccoli, spinach and collards), whole grain cereals,[2] and B complex vitamins with biotin and riboflavin. Vitamins C and E encourage good circulation. Rather than overload your body with supplements, check with a nutritionist or doctor to see what your body needs. Excessive sugar, salt, alcohol and caffeine are not good for the hair.[3]

Vitamins and minerals cannot correct poor hair conditions caused by underlying medical problems.

Maintenance

Oil treatments and weekly conditioning with products that contain healthy boosters restore the natural moisture level. These processes are especially important if the hair has been permed, frosted or bleached.

Buy products for your type of hair (dry, normal, oily) and condition (permed, frosted or treated). More and more hair care companies are using natural ingredients that come from the sea, plants, fruits and flower extracts. European women have a long tradition of using plants and herbs on hair and skin. Women who worry about multisyllabic chemicals may wish to investigate products that have ingredients they recognize.

If a hairdresser does your hair, express an interest in the products. Are they formulated for your hair type? Does he/she condition your hair after shampooing?

Cleansing. Even hair that has not been permed or bleached is damaged by harsh shampoos or soaps. Protein-rich shampoos protect the hair and keep it from looking drab. Before shampooing, massage your scalp to circulate the oil sitting on the skin.

Problem hair can frequently be traced to improper shampooing. This method keeps you from botching it.

1. Don't punish your hair with hot water! Wet hair thoroughly with warm water. Pour the shampoo into your palm, rub hands together and massage it into the scalp. If you need more lather, add a little water rather than more shampoo.

2. Rinsing is very important. Rinse three to four times longer than you shampoo to remove every trace of lather.

3. Condition after every shampoo.

4. Using cool water for the final rinse flattens the hair shaft, which promotes shine, and is invigorating.

5. Be gentle with wet hair. Pat dry to prevent breakage.

Conditioning. Conditioning after every shampoo with a protein-packed product restores elasticity, lost moisture and oils. This is essential for most women over 50. Because of stress, chemical processing, and environmental aggressions, the scope of conditioners has expanded from the ends of the hair only to formulations for both the hair and scalp. Some are pH balanced, 100% oil free, and dermatologist tested. Extra mild conditioners are available when frequent shampooing is necessary.

The functions of conditioners are to:

■ Replenish the moisture balance

■ Protect from damaging elements such as the weather and sun

■ Repair frequently styled, permed or color treated hair

- Add body to limp, fine or thinning hair

- Increase the shine, vitality and manageability without relaxing the curl

- Neutralize unwanted yellowing from grey and white hair.

Therapeutic conditioners specifically created for fragile African-American hair that breaks easily are available.

The labeling on the product describes its purpose. Excellent conditioners are found in the grocery stores, drugstores and beauty salons.

Don't over-condition. Too much of a good thing is just that—too much. Follow the directions on the package. A lot can be learned by talking with knowledgeable consultants in salons and beauty schools.

Hair Spray, Mousse and Gels. Use alcohol- and fragrance-free products that do not dull or dry and give control without stickiness. Some have sunscreen protection. Sprays with good holding power can be used for styling. After spraying, use a hair pick to lift, heighten, smooth or separate. Then, spray once more to set. Try this: shake your head while spraying to get that free-flowing feel.

Mousse is lightest hold, sprays are thicker and gels strongest. Use gel where you need extra body or hold and on damp, not soaking wet, hair. Too much of either product weights hair down.

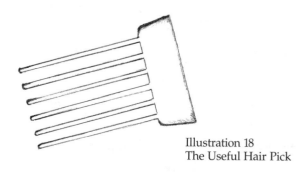

Illustration 18
The Useful Hair Pick

Dull-looking Hair. Shine lessens because the sebaceous glands produce less and less oil. Proper rinsing as already described is one factor for improvement. A lemon juice rinse brightens but is also drying. Some conditioners have natural ingredients such as rose essence to improve sheen. Look for hair sprays, rinses, shampoos and conditioners that add luster. Warm oil treatments are excellent all-around conditioners. Here's a basic recipe:

■ Heat olive, sesame or coconut oil to warm not hot.

■ Distribute evenly with a wide-toothed comb or your fingers from scalp to the ends.

■ Cover with thin plastic then wrap around with a towel that has been saturated in hot water and rung out.

■ Leave on 15 minutes, then shampoo, lathering twice. RINSE THOROUGHLY.

Fine and Thin Hair. Fine hair refers to the diameter of each strand that is so small the hair is limp. Thin refers to the number of hairs, which usually decreases with age. If your hair is thinning more than you like, you may wish to consult a dermatologist. Minoxidil is a prescription drug that gives impressive results.

Massaging to increase circulation, proper shampooing, conditioning and products specifically marked for fine and thin hair are all helpful. Products with body-building ingredients like panthenol and biotin (vitamin B factors), collagen (a form of protein), and magnesium add volume.

Bleaching or permanent coloring and fine-hair body perms create thicker hair and consequently more manageability by opening the cuticle and creating a fatter shaft. Extra curly perms clump strands together, making the hair look even less full. A chic short cut gives a neater, thicker look and does not weight fine hair down the way longer length does.[4]

Perming. Better products are constantly coming on the market. Your hairdresser should use the best ones for your type of hair. Too much chemical processing will dry and dull hair and can create problems. If you color, perm only if it is absolutely necessary. When it is, wait at least two to three weeks before coloring. Think in terms of a body wave for extra fullness no more than twice a year, preferably in the spring and fall. If you only need a touch-up for a place where you need more curl or wave, then, go for a spot perm.

The Curling Iron. Decades ago women would heat the curling iron in the gas flame of the stove, wetting their finger and quickly touching the iron to sizzle test its temperature. Today the iron comes in various sizes and heats up in seconds with temperature controls. It is still useful to bend, curl or wave stubborn hair.

> Dry hair? Try an overnight olive oil "bath." Pour on enough oil to saturate and finger comb from roots to tips. Sleep on a towel-covered pillow. Shampoo and rinse well to remove all oil.

Color

As the years go by, both the skin and hair lose coloring. The combination of a pale complexion with lightening hair makes us look older. Tinting the hair, makeup colorings and adorning the figure with a rainbow of richer clothing colors add vitality to the whole appearance.

Nature's rule is the more facial lines and/or wrinkles the lighter the color of the hair. If you're unhappy with greying hair, color it. Grey or white hair on women whose skin has yellow undertones is aging, but on women with blue undertones, it is attractive providing the grey or white is not dull or yellowish. If it is, look for shampoos, conditioners or rinses specifically for grey or white hair that remove the yellow or brassy tone and add a silvery luster. Drugstores and salons carry these.

The following are hair colors appropriate for the blue and yellow undertones of the skin:

Blue (cool undertones)	Yellow (warm undertones)
Ash blonde	Golden blonde
Silver grey and white	Flaxen blonde
Ash brown	Golden brown
Blue black and blue brown	Red brown

If you have fair skin, be careful about dark hair colors. The darker shades emphasize facial lines unless you have the right cosmetic shades and know how to use them with the darker hair. You may choose an all-over or partial coloring. Women with sensitive skin, or those who do not want chemicals on the scalp, find it advantageous to partially color or frost the hair. With this process the hair is pulled through a cap that prevents the chemical solution from touching and possibly traumatizing the scalp. Highlighting the hair around the temples uplifts droopy eyes and minimizes facial lines.

Color shampoos and mousses add color that lasts from shampoo to shampoo. The effectiveness of some of these products depends upon the porosity of the hair, its ability to absorb the color. Chemically treated hair i.e. permed or bleached has more porosity. Bleaching swells the hair shaft and gives it more body, more manageability. Women who

---

Look good coming and going. Fuss
with the front AND back of your hair.

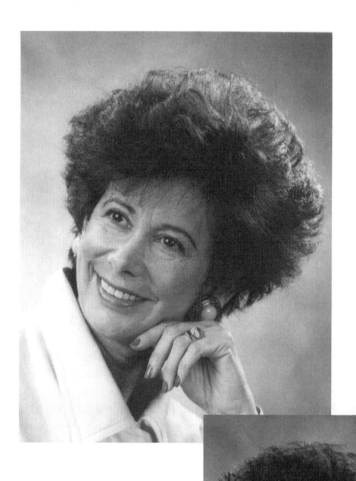

"The woman, not the years,
is the focus of my designs."
Hair and Makeup by Designer
Angela Grandinetti, Hair Cartel in Denver, CO

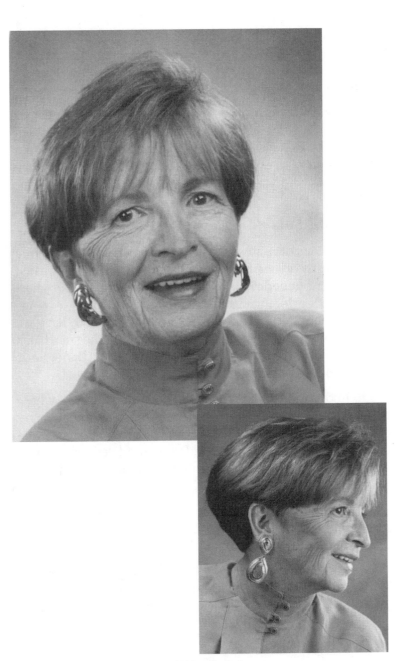

Hair and Makeup by Designer
Angela Grandinetti, Hair Cartel in Denver, CO

have colored their hair for years still maintain healthy-looking tresses because they nourish the hair on the outside, the body on the inside and participate in a body-moving activity to increase the circulation.

A friend was approaching her seventies and felt uncomfortable about her white hair so she had it colored pale golden blonde and was amazed at how much better she looked. At a family reunion, many of her relatives said she seemed to be the only one who wasn't getting older!

"How Do I Find a Good Hairdresser?"

Hair salons have shown little ingenuity in creating unique and individual styles for women over fifty. As we get older, they have one generic hairdo—teased or fluffed all over, short in back with a forehead curl here or there. This is okay for some women, but for all of us? On the other hand, have we been content with the same old styles thinking the smart look is not for us? Well, it is. Besides, a new, chic hairstyle is wonderful for the morale.

To find a good stylist, ask women—even strangers whose hairstyle you admire—who does their hair. Call the manager of a beauty school. They get lots of feed-back. Watch newspaper ads, or consult the Yellow Pages and telephone several salons in a location convenient to you. Make a short list of questions such as:

"Do you have an operator that is especially good at styling hair for women over 50? I would like something different and more up-to-date."

If they hem and haw over this question, cross them off your list. The way they respond tells a lot. You do not want a hairdresser who has out-dated misconceptions of how our hair should look.

"My hair is greying and I think it makes me look old. Do you have an experienced colorist who can advise me as to whether I should color my hair?"

If you want coloring, cutting and styling, speak to the manager of the shop to find out who is proficient in all three.

How to Work with a Hairdresser to Get the Best Hair Results

How many times have you come home from the hairdresser and recombed your hair? Seldom do stylists consider the overall appearance and personality before they take the scissors. Telling them a little about your lifestyle and showing pictures of hairstyles you like helps considerably. This is more effective than groping for the right words to describe something you may not be too sure of.

Before going to the salon, scan magazines, especially *Lears* and *Town and Country,* fashion brochures, even television, for hairstyles you would like to imitate. Collect pictures of the ones you like; the age of the woman in the photo is unimportant, only the hair. Don't get bogged down in analyzing whether a style will look right on you. That comes during your consultation with the hairdresser when you discuss whether a certain style, variation, or combination would be flattering for you. Right now you need several illustrations of what you like.

The best hair design is determined by the contours of the head, face, figure, and your personality. For example:

- If your nose is prominent, you need fullness at the back of the head.

- Bangs balance a high or broad forehead and focus attention on the eyes.

- Wear short hair for a short neck and longer hair for the longer neck.

- Hair on sides should have a combined width no greater than the width of your face.

- The height of your hair should not exceed the length of your forehead.

- If you are large-boned, tall or broad shouldered, your hair should be full, not skimpy, to balance the proportion of your figure. Conversely, if you are petite, your style needs to be closer to the head and slightly higher on top.

- Usually, the athletic woman may not care to look like a *grande dame de Paris.* She is more comfortable with an easy-to-care-for style as is the very busy woman.

Hair that is too long, too curly, too bouffant, too set is too aging. The lines of our hairstyles require movement. A gamin-type haircut—close-cropped in back, straight at the sides with straight bangs—may have been charming for years, but when facial lines and shadows become noticeable, this cut draws attention to them. The severity of extremes on most of us emphasizes facial lines. Instead, go for flowing softness.

Although short hair downplays aging, it is not for everyone. Some women will never wear it. A woman I know who is well over 80 has an abundance of shiny, snow-white, softly waving hair that is shoulder-length. This style perfectly fits her slim figure, throat, and personality.

Change is scary. That may be why we stick with one style. Many times we hesitate to voice our fears and then wonder why we don't get what we want. Discuss your ideas with the hairdresser, so he/she understands you better. Treat them as an interested friend. Then, don't snooze off. Pay attention to what is done. If they start to tease (also called back comb) your hair and you don't want teasing, say so, and it can easily be smoothed out. Hairdressers tease the hair to give it more body but if a body-building shampoo and conditioner are used, it is unnecessary. If they don't have these products, bring your own.

If you are unhappy with the results, say so before getting out of the chair. Feel comfortable saying, "I don't like the way my hair curls here" or "Can the color be softened?" Be specific. Don't be a cranky critic. That's counter-productive, but you do need to establish an intelligent relationship through honest dialogues. At the same time, say what you do like.

Conscientious hairstylists take pleasure in an artistically styled hairdo. They enjoy a woman who is interested in her appearance. If you are puzzled about how to get the same results after you leave their skillful fingers, ask how you can work with your hair between appointments. It's good advertising for them if your hair is attractive and easy to care for. A contented customer is a valuable asset, and so is a good hairdresser.

Shaping the Hair

Great hairdos start with good haircuts. When the cut still brushes into shape after three weeks, you know you've had a good one. Hair looks best and is easier to care for when it is trimmed every six to eight weeks.

Hair is shaped to balance and harmonize with the shape of the face. To do this, the hair should fluff out at the narrowest part of the face and be closer to the head at the widest. The following guidelines illustrate how to shape the hair according to the shape of the face:

Oval Face. This shape is enhanced with a simple hairstyle, slightly wavy in proportion to the face. Hair looks best

---

A quick and easy hairfix: Brush hair head-down and spray if you want more fullness. When you raise your head, smooth, shape and spray to set.

when worn away from the face. Off-center styles break the regular lines. Fullness at the sides can make the face seem long and narrow.

Thin Face. Curls, fullness and highlights at the sides make this face appear wider and more oval (see Illustration 19).

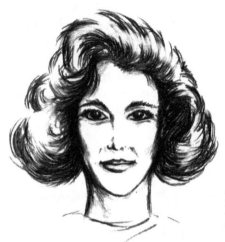

Illustration 19
Hair Shape for
a Thin Face

Triangular Face. Style hair close to the head at the widest part of the face and full at the narrowest part. Direct waves and curls towards the narrowest part.

1. Narrow at cheeks and brows, wider at chin and jawbone, pear-shaped: A center or low side part adds width to the brows. At the forehead add soft irregular, non-uniform bangs that flare out at each side, or gentle wisps of hair. Pulling the hair back from the forehead and temples is not flattering. Cut hair to earlobes or slightly above.

2. Inverted triangle, heart-shaped. Broad forehead with narrow jawline: Wear hair close to the head around the forehead and temples with a high side part and waves or wispy bangs. Let it be fuller from eyes to chin, neck and shoulder areas. Do not cut hair shorter than the bottoms of the earlobes (see Illustration 20).

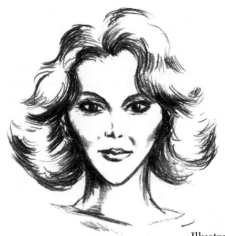

Illustration 20
Hair Shape for
Inverted Triangle Face

Narrow Chin. Wear hair a little below the ears with fullness or curls at jawline to balance receding jaw or pointed chin (see Illustration 21).

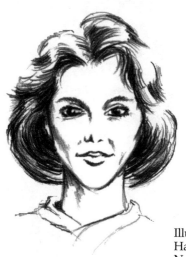

Illustration 21
Hair Shape for
Narrow Chin

Round Face. Cut the hair to the bottom of the earlobes with height and width on top and a high side part. Soft waves or curls toward the center of the crown gives needed height. Add highlights at the top. Sides should wave back and up. Longer hair should surround the face with curls/waves concentrating on the jaw, neck or shoulder area.

Square Face. An off-center part or soft, curly bangs swept to the sides soften the wide brow. Brush sides toward the face with volume above the forehead with gentle waves flowing back. Keep the hair styled close to the head at wide cheekbones. Straight hair and straight bangs do not flatter.

Wide Chin or Jaw. Keep hair short. Use soft curls/waves and fullness at the sides to balance out the strong chin.

Long Face. Wear a medium length, full not flat on the sides. Straight hanging hair makes your face seem drawn. Break the long line with curls and layering, and soft bangs for the high forehead (see Illustration 22). A colorful braided or full-bodied scarf, worn bandanna-like, flattens the crown, giving the illusion of width.

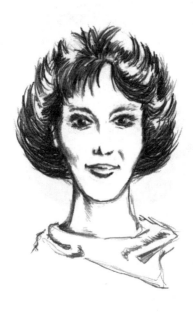

Illustration 22
Hair Shape for
Long Face

Low Forehead. Avoid bangs; use soft fullness above the forehead and at the crown to lengthen the forehead. Add highlights around the front of the hairline.

Wigs

"I can't think of any negatives about them!" enthused a wig-wearing woman. "They feel comfortable, look as good as my real hair and require minimal styling. They're fantastic!" and she wear wigs at least 40 hours every week. After discovering she had cancer and, before chemotherapy began, she bought two wigs, one the same color as her hair and the other a mix of lighter shades. Many people told her they couldn't see any difference between the wigs and her real hair.

Another woman, who was 20 years older, developed a disease of the scalp resulting in hair loss and caused by too much perming and coloring. Under the care of a dermatologist, she faithfully follows a remedial routine, and her hair is growing back (as is the first woman's). But in the meantime, she has four wigs and loves wearing them. The one she likes most is golden brown. To enhance it with a touch of naturalness she combs a little of her grey hair into the extra hair around her forehead. When wearing this wig, people have told her she looks 20 years younger.

Both women say they are not conscious of having a wig on; they are ultra lightweight. The second woman said the money she saves in shampoos, sets and cuts for two months equals the cost of one wig. The working woman buys wigs for convenience and others buy them for fun and fashion. Here are some tips:

1. When you go shopping for a wig, take a friend along (a must) and try to find an understanding, knowledgeable salesperson either in a wig shop or department store, who takes a personal interest in you, not just in making a sale.

2. Color is very important. The right color beautifies your your complexion and brings out the color of your eyes.

You may choose true-to-life shades or an alluring change, human hair or synthetic.

3. Expect some frustration in finding the right one. Don't buy on the first visit because the trying-on process is tiring. Try on several and then come back when you are refreshed. Check the wig's color in daylight because the light in stores is frequently deceptive.

4. Once you start wearing a wig, go without it as often as you can. Air is important to the growth of new hair.

5. For women who have lost or are losing their hair, acquire two or three turbans for wig-free time. They are available where you make your purchase or in Accessories at department stores.

Wigs are full of promise with impressive possibilities for women who are devastated by thinning hair, who want the convenience and time-saving advantages, and for women who fancy an exciting change just for the fun of it.

7

Fashion for Your Figure

"You can look smashing, no matter
what size and shape you are."
—Barbara Weiland and
Leslie Wood[1]

No body is perfect! And no amount of exercise or dieting alters your basic body structure. When weight change is impossible, accept the way you are, and spend your energy drawing attention to the best features and de-emphasizing the not-so-good ones. The following elements of design are basic to enhancing and camouflaging:

Line. Vertical lines in the cut of the garment and the use of color add length to your figure; horizontal lines in the cut and print of the fabric add width.

Color. The smart use of color creates optical illusions, making the figure appear bigger, thinner or more perfect than it is. Monochromatic outfits and one-color apparel slenderize. Use light and bright colors to accent your best features; darker or neutral ones play down the pounds or minimize unattractive proportions. White gives a bigger look and if worn around the face it can drain color from the complexion, showing up lines and shadows.

Textures of Fabrics. Fuzzy, tweedy and shiny fabrics give the illusion of adding weight to the figure. Shiny fabrics and soft textures around the throat are a flattering frame for the face. Smooth, fine knits accent contours more than those with a nap like boucles or nubby weaves. Wearing contrasting textures such as a cashmere sweater with a silk skirt smack of sublime style. Natural materials—cotton, wool, silk, linen— have an easy simplicity that wears well in all seasons. Resiliency is often improved when the natural fibers are combined with synthetics.

Body Types

It's an easy art to give good proportion to the various body types. By camouflaging the negatives we give good form to the figure. A combination of two or more of these body types applies to most women. Few of us fit completely into one category. When you know your body type, shopping is simplified.

Evenly Proportioned/Average Height. With balanced proportions, you can wear color a variety of ways. Bright colors enlarge, so if this is not a problem, use them to enhance your best features. Analyze your figure and use vertical lines where you wish to slenderize and horizontals where you need more fullness or width.

Triangle/Narrow at Shoulders with Larger Hips and Legs. With large hips choose jackets that are hip- or thigh-length. Keep bright colors and interest items above the waist; wear subdued or darker shades below. Draw attention up with ropes of beads or shiny metals.

The additional width of shoulder pads trim the waist and hip line, improving upper body proportions. Padding should conform to the bone structure with subtle extension (see Illustration 23). Padding that is obviously bulky or extends too far beyond the shoulder line overpowers upper body proportions, particularly if you are under five feet four inches. An undergarment with padding, for example a chemise with built-in pads, adds smoother construction to the hang of your clothing than some garments with pads attached. Clip-on pads that give curvy or square shapes are also available.

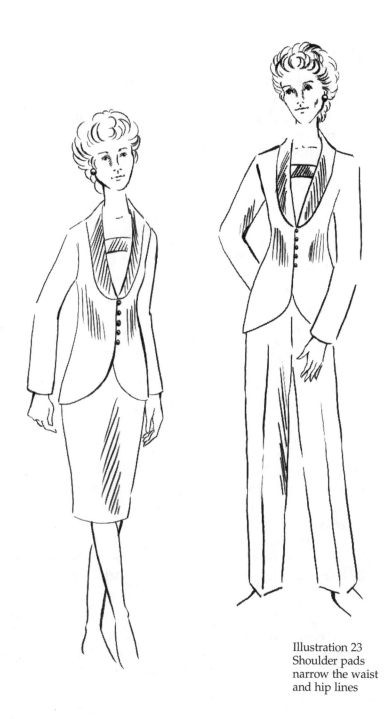

Illustration 23
Shoulder pads
narrow the waist
and hip lines

Super-long, super-sleek separates create a slimmer look as do man-tailored slacks with room at the top. Be careful with pleats. If the silhouette is too baggy, you'll look hippy. Inverted pleats are best (see Illustration 24). Let trousers fall straight with no flap around the ankles. If you are five feet four inches or under, the cuffless hem gives the longer line. Mid-calf pants balance wide hips.

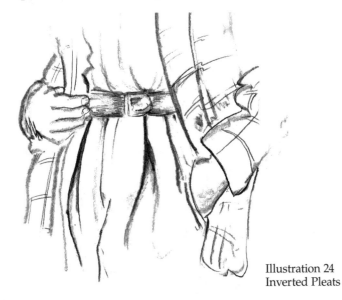

Illustration 24
Inverted Pleats

Use simple, slightly flared skirts with less fabric but not too tight at the hipline. Long narrow skirts in solid colors with matching hose and shoes are slimming. Gathered skirts add pounds to the hips. Wear skirts that flair below the hips with sweaters, shirts and overblouses that go down to the point where the flair begins. Patch pockets on the hips and wide belts make hips look wider. Narrow belts are appropriate.

Inverted Triangle/Wide Shoulders, Narrow Torso. Use subdued colors on upper body with a dark tailored jacket and matching skirt or slacks. Color on pockets at hipline add width to the narrow part of your figure. Bright colors are best worn below the waist. Man-style shirts in crisp fabrics and oversize sweaters and dresses without shoulder pads will not give a top heavy look. Be wary of pads that do. Skirts with pleats or flair balance the wide shoulder line.

Plump or Overweight. Vertical panels of color from shoulders to hemline slenderize, for example, a two-toned suit with one side of the jacket in a neutral, the other side, a darker color. Stay away from horizontal lines and plaids. Use bright colors for small accents.

Rather than contrasting colors such as a white blouse with black slacks, try monochromatic combinations i.e. pearl grey blouse with slacks or skirt in a darker grey or vice versa, depending upon the proportions of your figure. One-color and monochromatic dressing for the large woman creates the illusion of tall and trim. Fake out fat with long uninterrupted lines such as vertical ribbing and generously cut cable knits or cardigans with the plunging neckline.

Go for oversized sweaters and overblouses with simple skirts or straight-leg (no flair) slacks. Acid-wash jeans add pounds as do dirndl skirts. Skirts with deep pleats or gathers make even a slim figure look chunky. Dresses may blouse above waist to balance hips. Depending on your height, keep hems just below knees or mid-calf. No matter how big your frame is, shoulder pads square the upper body giving the illusion of narrowing the hip area—an important factor for this body type.

Wear only your most flattering colors and fabrics that move with simple, fluid lines like fine knits, lightweight cottons, soft cashmeres and silks; or, try linens, crisp cottons and gabardines if they fit your style and slenderize. Tight fits outline bulges.

Too Thin. One woman said, "Everyone talks about women who are too fat, what about people like me who are too thin?" You can use the opposite of everything described for the plump figure, adapting the dressmaking lines and color design to your height and the proportions of your figure. Prints with dominant horizontal lines, bright and contrasting colors, fitted jackets, textured fabrics, big knits, full, flowing skirts and pleated slacks can all be in your closet.

Five Feet Seven Inches and Over. Wear contrasting colors, top and bottom. Interrupt one-color outfits with a contrasting color in belt or peplin. Use color interest in large handbags, jewelry and accessories. Horizontal lines and plaids balance with your height. Wear jackets that come below the hipline. For slacks, pleats are fine if you are not too hippy, and so are cuffs. For large hips, slacks with straight lines look best.

Summer-cool loose, full pants or skirts are lovely on the taller figure if they are cut in body-conscious ways and/or sharpened with graphic prints.

Under Five Feet Four Inches—Petite. Try vertical lines in the color, print and cut of apparel. No belt unless you wear shoes with higher heels. Belts of the same fabric or same color do not interrupt the one-color line as much as those in a contrasting color do. Wear your hemline barely below the knees or floor length. If you are long-waisted, wear jackets or sweaters that come to the hips or a little below. Cuffless, tapered slacks give a longer line.

Camouflaging Figure Challenges

The basic rules are:

- To de-emphasize, use dark or neutral colors;
- To slenderize, wear vertical lines in color and style, and monochromatic combinations (see Illustration 25);
- To widen or add pounds, use horizontal lines in the cut of the garment and in color with light, bright shades.

> Fashion choices depend upon figure proportions.

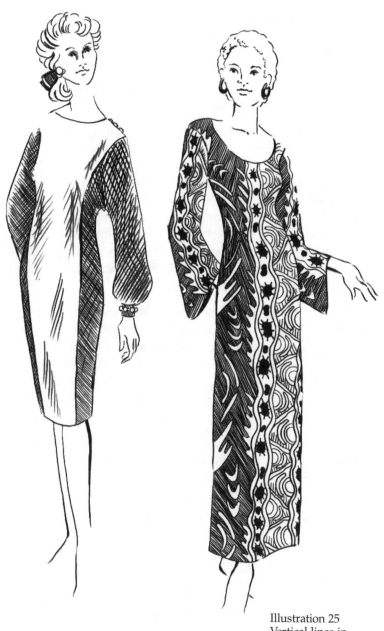

Illustration 25
Vertical lines in
cut, color and design
slenderize.

Sagging Bosoms. Nothing ages a figure more than breasts that droop. A supportive bra restores a firmer, higher silhouette. Generally, the point of the bosom should be four to six inches below the armpit, depending on the structure of your body. The uplifted bust line balances your figure and corrects the matronly look.

When I mentioned improving the bust line in a Glamour for Grandmas class, the women couldn't resist covertly scanning everyone's chest. Suddenly, one woman blurted out, "My, yours sure look good!" We followed her gaze to Ann, whose trim sweater revealed a teen-like bustline. "Well, they should," she said with a note of satisfaction. "This is a $500 bra!" To answer our astonishment, she explained she had had a double mastectomy. "Ever since I was in my high school, my pendulous breasts were burdensome and embarrassing. Now I can look the way I want to!"

Full Bust. Use shallow V-necks, the shawl neckline, or convertible and open collars at the throat. Cardigan and Chanel jackets, and A-line, shift and shirt-waist styles are good. No gaping button fronts! Remedy by inserting gussets under the arms. Quilted, embroidered, beaded, sequined or studded details in the shoulder area of a garment or a large colorful broach/pin on this upper line draws the gaze up.

For the woman who participates in body-jerking activities like jazzercise, fast walking or tennis, the knitted, elasticized sports bra gives the confidence of needed support.

Heavy Upper Arms. No strapless, sleeveless fashions or skinny knit sleeves. Opt for the full-cut sleeves i.e. dolmen or kimono. Sleeves can be rolled to the elbows but keep them loose-fitting.

Stooped Shoulders/Rounded Back. Shirt collars are better than jewel necklines. Big soft scarves flatter, not narrow skimpy ones. Avoid fabrics that cling to the upper body. Go for fabrics with texture—boucle, fuzzy, nubby—rather than flat knits. Allow blouses and jackets to be full across the back of the throat and have enough body to hang straight. No belts. You can visualize how a fitted garment accentuates contours. The same applies to coats.

For an additional lift, brush hair away from your face and throat and in the back, cultivate a soft, swept-up short coiffure. Avoid straight severe cuts.

No Waistline. Don't wear belts on anything, not even coats. Wear straight lines, shoulders to hips, and no one will know your waist size. An exceptionally well-groomed woman I know is 5'2", slightly over-weight with no waist, yet people were always complimenting her on what she wore and asking her advice. She honed her skill to camouflage an imperfect figure so effectively that the "limitations" were never obvious. She had no special training, but thoughtfully observed, compared, analyzed and enjoyed designing and redesigning her clothes.

Plump Mid-Section. The paunch is a familiar problem. Here are some ways to conceal it:

1. Use darker shades below the waist.

2. One-color outfits without belts minimize.

3. Avoid fitted clothing and clingy fabrics.

4. Shirt-waist dresses with straight lines, fullness above and below the waist flatter. Peplums and drop-waist dresses work, too.

5. Roomy, not sloppy, jackets, vests, overblouses, and long sweaters conceal. If you are tall or long-waisted, these garments may come to or below the hip line.

6. Color accents around the throat and shoulders draw attention away from the torso as do interesting necklines designed with scarves or jewelry.

7. Bolder shoulders take inches off the midsection.

8. Be wary of gathered or full-pleated skirts, especially if you are under 5'3". They often make even a slim figure appear chunky.

9. Never buy pocketless side-zip jeans—they make the bulge more prominent as do jeans that are too tight. Keep them loose-fitting with front pleats or a V-seamed front yoke (see Illustration 26).

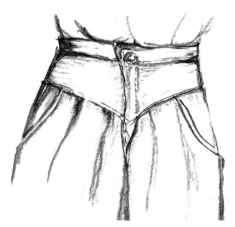

Illustration 26
The V-seamed Yoke

10. Girdles are not what they used to be. Lightweight and tissue-thin, they are machine washable, spun in spandex and nylon, providing good control without the consciousness of wearing one. Some have a high waist to smooth out the mid-section roll. The all-in-one combination of bra and girdle, is another comfortable and firming alternative.

Extra Weight on Outer Thighs. Sleek straight, long lines are slimming. Pleats in slacks should not be too full. Let them taper to the ankles—no flapping hems. If hips are wide, too much taper creates a balloon effect. Stretchy fabrics exaggerate contours as do mottled acid-wash jeans. Uniform color is as slimming as a diet.

Broad Hips. The hem of a jacket should be above the widest part of the hips if you are short waisted. The longer jacket provides flattering coverup. One-color outfits and darker tones below the waistline will de-emphasize. Front pockets on trousers draw attention to this area; slash pockets are better.

Heavy and Thin Legs. Slacks with deep pleats fall smoothly over heavy legs and camouflage thin ones. Clinging fabrics add pounds and draw attention to bulges.

Light colored hose fill out the thin legs and darker shades slim down the heavier ones.

For slender legs, slim skirts that come to or below the knee cover the thinner thigh while showing off the shapeliest part of your legs, the calves. Avoid A-line and full skirts, and bulky fabrics like tweedy wools and wide-wale corduroys that make thin legs look stick-like. If you want a long, full skirt, select one in a soft, flowing fabric—rayons, silks, cotton knits—with flat or low-heeled shoes. High heels with any skirt make legs look thinner.

Hemline. Generally, hemlines should be worn at the knee or lower, depending on your height. Be sure the hem does not stop at the heaviest part of your legs. Wear it either higher or lower.

———————

Make a checklist of the flattering fashion factors for your figure and keep them in mind when you shop. It simplifies selection.

Women over fifty have graduated beyond fads, mini-skirts and bikinis. Still they are fun-loving and feel years and sometimes decades younger than their age. They want their image to reflect that feeling with wardrobe selections tailored to interests and activities in fabric textures and styles lines that feel good on the body—apparel that is adaptable to different climatic conditions indoors as well as out, easy to pack and practical for travel.

Shop Like a Professional

- Don't shop when you're hurried, hungry, tired or moody. You'll buy on impulse just to get relief.

- If the budget is tight and a special occasion is coming up, you may not need a new head-to-toe outfit. Instead, why not get a new accessory or two?

- Don't buy anything too tight. You may not lose 5 pounds!

- Don't buy slacks without the sit/bend test or you may have to stand up in them.

- New technology is improving the quality of synthetics. Good polyester charmeuse beats poor quality silk. Search for blends in which the natural fiber dominates.

- Best buys are made of year-round fabrics such as silk, viscose, wool and cotton. Versatile blends with natural fibers are cool in summer and can be layered in winter.

- Two color outfits never fail. If a third color comes into play, it's a neutral—white, grey, beige, brown, navy or black.

- Judge clothes by the fit, not the size on the tag. Check out the front, back AND side view. Try on as many sizes as necessary to get a good fit. Sometimes the cut of the garment, not the size, poses a problem.

- Before you buy, ask yourself: Do I have the body for this fashion? Does it go with at least two other items I already have? Think simplicity, ease, comfort, color.

- Look for details that indicate quality: fine-tooth zippers in neat plackets; bound buttonholes; shoulder pads that follow the lines of your body, neither too full or too extended.

- Don't let sales people seduce you into compromising your taste.

- Discount fashion stores and near-new shops have some excellent merchandise at big savings.

- Avoid feeling indebted to helpful salespeople. Just because they looked for your size in the stock room, you don't have to buy it.

- P.T. Barnum said there's a sucker born every minute. Don't be taken in by these classic come-ons:

  "You'll just have to buy that, it's you."

  "It's a different style, but you'll get used to it."

  "Oh, you can easily alter that."

  "It's the only one left in stock. I just can't keep them on the rack."

  "It looks great on you, and I wouldn't say that to every-one."

You are more important than your clothing. What you wear reflects your individuality and should not detract from the person you are. Color and design as well as fun and comfort are equally important. The ultimate test is: Does it make you feel happy and confident?

> With a positive attitude, the total glamour image is possible beyond 50 and beyond size 10.

8

Hands

...think of your nails as your
BEST accessory, like a beautiful
ring, bracelet or scarf."
—Patricia Bozic[1]

Hands are always on display and are very expressive. Whether they are wrinkled, spotted, veiny, scarred, or none of these—even with stubby nails—they look 100% better and younger when lubricated daily and manicured. With careful conditioning, the appearance of hands and nails improves in three to four weeks.

Adrien Arpel[2] suggests soaking hands in warm olive oil for a few minutes to soften the skin and strengthen the nails. For comfort and smoothness, cleanse hands with your facial cleanser, then use a facial mask on your hands and fingers. After rinsing, massage them with an emollient cream or oil. Starting at the finger tips, as though you were putting on kid gloves, rub down each finger from tip to joint, then from joints to wrist and last, the palms. Treat them with the same care that you give to your face.

> If you have to put your hands in water, add a couple tablespoons of vinegar to counteract dryness.

Easy Exercise for Flexibility _____

A one-minute daily routine invigorates, relieves stiffness, and adds flexibility and grace.

- Tightly clench fists then splay fingers stretching them out till you feel the stretch from palm to finger tips.

- Quickly, clench and stretch fingers five to eight times.

Considering all the work your hands have done and are doing, don't they deserve special treatment?

Spots, Scars or Vitiligo _____

Laser Treatments. A board certified (see pages 87, 88) plastic surgeon or dermatologist who specializes in the laser process for surface conditions performs these treatments on an outpatient basis. They painlessly and harmlessly remove age spots. Women have been very happy with the results.

Cosmetic Correctives. Covermark by Lydia O'Leary and Dermablend are available in department stores and drugstores. They come in different shades and are natural-looking, inexpensive cover-ups.

Self-Tanning Products. These oils, cremes or gels stain the skin, blending in with discolorations. Finding the color that goes with your skin may be tricky. Massage in with a circular motion when skin is warm and moist—preferably after a shower/bath. To prevent staining the fingers, wash them immediately after application. Reapply for deeper color. *Follow the directions on self-tanning products and cosmetic correctives.*

Manicure and polish nails with a stunning shade. Do this plus one of the three above, and your hands will look better than you ever believed possible.

Fingernails

The essentials to healthy nails are eating foods rich in protein, fats, minerals, carbohydrates and iron (i.e. fish, liver, oats, oranges, cauliflower, dried beans, leafy greens), vitamins B biotin and B_{12}, C, D, E, calcium with magnesium. Liver extract tablets have nutrients and other trace minerals that may help nails as well as hair and teeth. Elimination of toxins and good circulation are important.

Nails respond quickly to care. Nail abuse takes longer to correct. Hardeners, primers, base coats and top coats are effective against breakage. Polish reinforces enabling them to grow longer. Look for polishes with nail strengtheners and beneficial ingredients like aloe, keratin and protein.

Polish, lacquer, enamel are basically the same. Polish is not drying but the acetone in polish remover is. Use a non-acetone remover with moisturizing ingredients. High-priced polishes are not necessarily better than low-priced ones. Many contain formaldehyde which has been known to yellow and dry out nails, and its vapors may irritate the mucous membranes of the eyes, nose or mouth. Clinique and Almay now have enamels without formaldehyde, and the Lorik Nail System, available in salons and beauty supply stores, is formaldehyde-free and hypo-allergenic. With polishes that contains formaldehyde, use a formaldehyde-free base coat.

100 percent cotton balls and cotton pads absorb quickly, easily remove the polish, and do not leave residual fibers to show up under the polish. Skimpy synthetic puffs are not as absorbent. To save money buy a cotton roll from a drugstore and cut into workable pads.

The Easy Home Manicure

1. Scrub the nails with a soft brush, and soak in sudsy water to soften cuticles. Cuticle care is essential to strong nails.

2. Massage the cuticle area. Gently push back the cuticle around the moon with an orange stick or rubber-tipped

cuticle pusher. You can also do this while relaxing in the bathtub. Trim only when absolutely necessary because damaging cuticles can injure the growing nail plate and lead to infection. Nip away the rough dry skin on the sides. Apply a nail and/or cuticle conditioner, and if your nails are particularly dry, reapply. Applying a conditioner on the cuticle area is beneficial even when nails are polished.

3. Let nails dry completely before filing or they may split. Use an emery board and file gently, finishing by buffing the edges. Avoid filing deeply on sides where they are most vulnerable to be weakened. Round-shaped tips are easier to maintain and encourage better growth. To have the most elongated and balanced shape, file the nails to correspond with the outline of your cuticles. Keep all nails the same in length and shape (see Illustration 27).

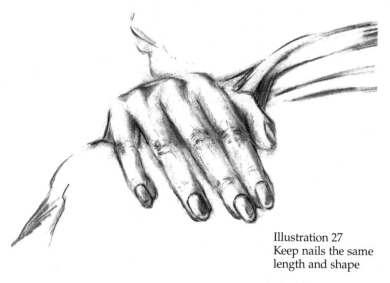

Illustration 27
Keep nails the same
length and shape

4. Buff lightly from the cuticles to tips until they are shiny. Avoid the feeling of friction or a burning sensation. Too much buffing wears down the surface of the nails. A three-way buffer, available in beauty supply stores, gives a sheen comparable to clear nail polish.

5. When nails are dry and free of oil, brush on a base coat—a ridge-filling base if you have bumpy nails or a nail-hardening base coat to fortify soft or weak nails. A base prevents staining, allows uniform application of nail color and "anchors" the lacquer so that it lasts longer.

6. To polish the nails—

   ■ Brush down the center of the nail first then each side.

   ■ Let the first coat dry, then apply the second. Two thin coats gives even color and the polish lasts longer.

   ■ Apply a top coat or sealer. For more durability stroke it under the tips. To prevent chipping, topcoat tips frequently.

   It usually takes about four hours for polish to dry hard. To expedite the drying process:

   ■ Use a fast drying top coat or nail polish;

   ■ Dip nails in ice cold water for about 30 seconds; or

   ■ Spray with a commercial product specifically for quick drying.

A manicure is a relaxing routine, easily done during a television program, listening to the radio or while reading a book. The resulting beauty confidence is well worth it. Let the nails go bare a day or two. Re-treat, reshape, and massage cuticles. Repair chips by simply recoloring and topcoating.

Warm temperatures thicken nail colors. Keeping them in a small caddy in the refrigerator prevents this. You can thin thickened polish by adding a few drops of nail polish solvent, available in a drugstore.

How to Choose Colors

Choose nail colors according to your preference, wardrobe colors and your skin tone. With the exception of brown or black skin, avoid burgundies, maroons and browns because they are aging to the skin. Most women can wear a true red. Nail color does not have to match your lips, but the shades should harmonize. Neutrals, light beiges, natural pinks, corals, and classic reds are versatile enough to go with everything, and the paler shades don't show chipping.

Colors Look Darker in the Bottle _____

If your hands are...	Use
Ruddy	Clear red, pink-based coral, soft pink and rose. No oranges.
Milky white, translucent	Soft pastels, mauve, plum, neutrals or the French manicure (tips only in beige-white, covered with a clear glaze).
Olive-toned	Blue-reds such as raspberry, cherry and burgundy.
Brown or black	Vivid shades, rich berries, wine, fuchsia, burgundy.
Tanned	Hot pinks, corals, orange-reds, frosts.
Small	Bright colors.
Visible Veins	Avoid blue-reds; they make veins more noticeable.
Bony	Muted colors.
Sallow or faded tan	Vivid shades.
Short, thick fingers	Flesh tones, neutrals.
Wide nails	Two shades same family; apply darker shade to outsides and lighter shade to middle; or don't put color all the way to the sides.
Large	Dark shades

For sheer subtlety, look for the transparencies and opalescents, or frosted translucent shades with a whisper of color.

Patricia Bozic in *30 Days to Beautiful Nails* says, "Perhaps you consider your nails details and don't want to take the time to give them the care they need...Well-groomed nails make you feel prettier and more feminine...No matter what condition yours are in right now—red, ragged, ridged, split, cracked, or bitten to the quick—you can make them stronger and more beautiful by following a regular nail care regime."[3]

9

Accessories

"Accessories are the secret
ingredients to developing
[your] style."
—LeAnn L. Nelson[1]

Set off your fashion statement with an accessory to add a note of fun, zest or elegance. That could be jewelry, scarves, belts, shoes, hosiery or hats.

For the monochromatic outfit, accessories can be in the same color family or in sympathetic/complementing shades i.e. for a pink outfit use a contrasting black patent leather belt and pumps. When you combine a bold color and a neutral such as a cobalt blue and white suit, the accessories should pick up either or both of these colors, maybe cobalt-colored pumps and a white purse.

Choose accessories to play up your best features, for example, earrings that bring out the sparkle in your eyes; elaborate rings for attractive hands; pumps to flatter shapely legs.

All accessories should work with the contours of your body. If you have fleshiness around the throat or if your throat is short, wear necklines, scarves and jewelry at least four inches below the top of the collarbone to avoid the choked-up look. The longer throat can wear the beaded, velvet choker bands and scarves circling the throat with a pin or clip attached.

Jewelry. Large jewelry complements large features, but overpowers the smaller, more delicate face. One or two distinctive pieces are more elegant for special occasions than several. For a more casual look and occasion, wear a variety. Flashy costume pieces like twisted metallic ropes, glass jewels in a rainbow of precious or faux stones, or spiral bracelets make old clothing look new.

Whether to wear silver or gold depends on the skin tone and clothing colors. Some women can wear both silver and gold. Gold corresponds to the warm tones; silver, to the cool. Go for the fun of wearing a shiny gold or silver chain with a casual, even sporty, outfit.

Luminous pearls brighten the face and add personal charm for day and evening wear. Try two lengths, one short and one long, or combine with beads or scarves. Rhinestone and faceted-crystal necklaces brighten evening apparel. If the budget allows, acquire a couple fine pieces of quality jewelry. They give years of pleasure.

The possibility of losing expensive earrings lessens when you have pierced ears, and you can still wear clipons. Medium-to-large sized button earrings cover wrinkled lobes. Think twice about heavy hanging pierced earrings that pull ear holes down. They look strange, except in Africa.

Keep in mind that long earrings draw attention to the lower part of the face and the throat.

Who said earrings had to be identical? It might be better with asymmetrical hairstyles to have a bigger adornment on one ear than on the other. With multiple colors in dressing you may want earrings to pick up two of the colors.

Pins express your mood and individuality. Use them on hip pockets and belts or in clusters. A dramatic or heirloom piece placed near the shoulder dresses up a Chanel suit.

A geometrically-designed fabric can be accompanied with dissimilar shapes in jewelry. Innovation increases enjoyment in fashion.

Scarves. For decades, scarves have been the trademark of Sparky, a woman living in the rural country of Washington State. She has a couple dozen rectangular, circular and square scarves from many countries. With dresses, skirts and blouses she wears exotic ones. But for work she has color coded them for each task: yellow for mowing grass, blue for hen house cleaning, lavender for tidying the barn, red for picking berries, cerise for weeding—she hates weeding and loves pink, orange for sweeping the walks and porches, flamboyant pink for washing windows, and brown for working with the bees.

One morning she was wearing an old gray sweatshirt over pedal pushers accessorized with a varicolored green scarf covering curlers and a matching one around her throat, tied in back, the ends fluttering in the breeze as she pushed a wheelbarrow of horse droppings to nourish a flower garden. Her neighbor, a retired doctor, not a well man, smiled as he watched and leaned over the fence to say, "Sparky, it's amazing how charming you look when you're hauling manure. You always make me feel better when I see you in one of your beautiful scarves." With her mania for scarves, her husband thinks that somehow Sparky, now 80, always looks prettier than other women.[2]

Select these fun-filled accessories to pick up the colors of your clothing or to add a note of contrast. To be a true complement to your costume, they need to look like an integral part, not like an add-on or afterthought.

Chiffon, silk, and lightweight polyester textures in brights, pastels, neutrals or woven with sparkling threads are kind to the face. Try eye-catching scarves in paisleys,

---

If your scarf tends to wander from its best position, anchor it under your garment with a safety pin.

geometrics, florals or plaids. Printed scarves go with printed clothing as long as the colors are identical. For example, a scarf or tie splashed with red and white polka dots adds a jaunty touch to a red and white striped shirt or dress.

Try this graceful frame for the face. Use a large square sheer silk or chiffon scarf, fold into a triangle, and place around your throat. Pull the two ends of the long edge through a scarf clip. Place ends in back and adjust loose folds under chin or drape them over one shoulder. Wear over sweater, dress or with a jacket. You can also add glitter to the folds by wearing a necklace that picks up the colors of the scarf, chain(s) or pearls in a short length or longer.

Even more interesting is combining opposites—a silk chiffon scarf woven with a metallic thread over a casual knit, or a frothy lace scarf with a denim jacket and/or jeans.

For the sophisticated cavalier look, fold a silk scarf cravat-like inside an open-necked cotton shirt (see Illustration 28).

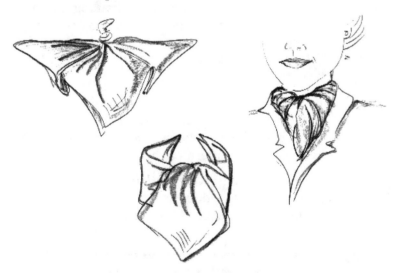

Illustration 28: Cravat Tie (medium size square scarf)
Gather up four or five inches of the center; tie in a knot; spread out like a diamond with the knot underneath; pick up two opposite corners and place around your throat, tie in back, tuck in knot.

Enfold your favorite long chain in a scarf as you drape it around your throat or waist.

When using a scarf for contrast or as an accent, let your lip color and nail polish pick up the accent color.

To cover the throat, wrap a small rectangular scarf around twice and tie in front or on the side. Fasten with your favorite clip or pin. The width of the scarf depends upon the length of your throat.

If you have a jacket with a low neckline, use it to showcase a flashy scarf and/or an heirloom pendant (see Illustrations 29, 30, 31).

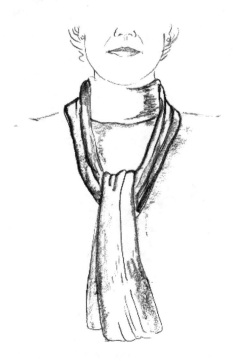

Illustration 29: Oblong Flip (36" or larger oblong scarf)
For added flair, embellish with a chain, pearls or beads.

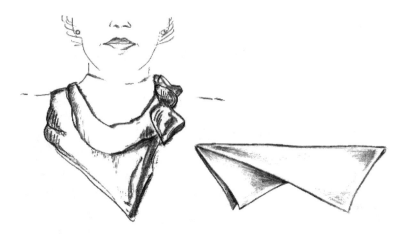

Illustration 30: Versatile Collar (36″ or larger square scarf)
Fold square in half to form a rectangle. Then fold diagonally to form
one straight edge and two points. Drape straight edge around shoulders.
Bring two ends of the straight edge together at front and tie in a square
knot—right over left then left over right. Wear with knot in front, on
shoulder or in the back.

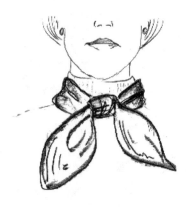

Illustration 31: Oblong Tie (short or long oblong scarf)
Tie a loose half knot at the place where you want the knot to appear
at the center of the throat. Bring the other end around the neck and pull
it through the loop of the knot. Adjust tightness.

Hats. Like scarves, hats need to complement the contours of your face and look like a matching part of your outfit in style, color and mood. To illustrate, please see the photograph on page 153.

Handbags. They don't have to match your shoes. The most popular choice is a quality handbag with lots of utilitarian pockets in a taupe, saddle brown or any versatile neutral that goes with everything. The size of the handbag reflects the size of the figure but many women opt for larger bags regardless. For special occasions, the shallow, small purse goes well with the petite figure and a larger bag for the woman who is over five-foot-five—and the more elegant the gown the simpler the bag.

Totes. Tote-toting women are happy women. They have everything their life depends upon in that wonderful tote, well, almost everything. Totes have become the essential accessory in an explosion of exciting patterns and compositions: plain canvas with bright trim; bold graphics on brilliant blue, black or red; a pageant of floral blossoms against pastels or white; giant daisies on brown; the posh one-color leather or exotic skins. Women are acquiring a wardrobe of totes to house their necessities and to go out and about with that wonderful feeling, "I have everything I need."

Hosiery. The one-tonal look from leg to foot is a slick, figure-flattering, pulled-together style. Or, match hem and hose, or hem, hose and shoes. Either way, color coordinating shoes with hose and hem, adds a touch of class. For seasonal harmony, go for the dark shoes with dark hose or lighter-colored shoes and hose. Deep-hued hosiery make legs look thinner, and the paler ones make them look fuller; and the more open the shoe, the sheerer the hose.

For shorts and short skirts and slicker-looking legs, wear pull-on tights or pantyhose. Match them to your outfit or select neutral tones. Control top pantyhose smooth out the tummy and cover the panty line under slacks.

A snazzy seventy-plus athlete race-walked in the Senior Games in a black hip-high body suit with suntan tights. When a friend admired her sylph-like figure, she said with a twinkle in her eyes, "I love tights. They sure do firm up the flab!"

Compatible Hose and Shoes

Shoes	Hose
Slip-ons or flats	Sheer or opaque
Oxfords	Bright or dark tones or the same color as shoes, and knit tights
Pumps	Opaque or sheer
Boots	Tights or hose to match the hem or boots

Shoes. Shoes are good updaters with a good fit and comfort being top priority. Scott Norman, a women's shoe salesman in New York City, recommends shopping for shoes in midafternoon because feet swell as the day goes on. Soft leather uppers mold to the irregularities of the foot. Leather soles conform better than non-leather, are lightweight, bend easier and, if stitched, indicate top quality.

The ever-smart spectator pumps are appropriate year-round in combinations such as taupe with black, black with brown, red with black, bluette with black, or cream (instead of white) with black. Stylish shoes now have comfortable heels. Silver and gold flats, loafers in luxury reptilian skins, suede and patent in multiple colors spruce up any outfit. Shoes in brilliant reds, emeralds, purples, turquoise or pastels give zing to your fashion statement and put spring in your step.

Accessories extend our wardrobe by creating the illusion of many different outfits. Besides this, they quicken interest, spice up style, and hint at individual uniqueness.

10

Coping with Defeminizing Surgery

I believe that it is possible to find
some joy in almost every experience...
What is a happy ending? Is it having
a face without wrinkles? Is it never
being ill or disappointed? Is it never
losing a loved one? I think not. For me,
a happy ending is the knowledge that,
even though the flame may flicker, my
inner candle of joy burns brightly.
—Lois Tschetter Hjelmstad
Fine Black Lines[1]

When I met the author of the above quote, her first words after the usual pleasantries were, "Why don't you write something for women like me?" Her book, *Fine Black Lines*, chronicles her life with cancer through journal entries, essays and poetry. Ever since she was a girl, she has used poetry to think through the gamut of her emotions. Cancer intensified that process, leaving her with a strong desire to help smooth the road for women like her.

Although this chapter refers to mastectomy and ostomy, I hope all women facing any kind of defeminizing surgery— and their friends and relatives—will be helped. My research reveals that practically everyone knows someone who has had or will have this experience.

Losing body parts is as traumatizing as losing a loved one. The mental pain is as acute as the physical and never completely goes away. But, the unbeatable human spirit marries disaster to progress, surmounts the tragic and challenges the impossible. Like all wise people, women who have had defeminizing surgery strive to get on with their lives and to stay on the lighter side as much as possible.

Even if women talk about their surgery of substraction—some cannot—we can barely understand the will and courage it takes for them to carry on. The majority find that maintaining a good appearance captures a firmer sense of normalcy. We are much more than the bland woman who looks back from the mirror in the morning. A positive, colorful image more clearly portrays our true personality, and living another day is a little easier. This is not pollyanna.

Self-esteem, confidence and the happiness quotient go up when a woman's reflection expresses the person she knows she is. That is a scientific fact, enunciated in the *Standard Textbook for Professional Estheticians* by Joel Gerson and *Psycho-Cybernetics* by Dr. Maxwell Maltz, a plastic surgeon. I have seen this hundreds of times in my classes.

The first women I talked with are in a cancer support group. They hunt for humor, squeeze joy and rewards from every day, and get together to laugh over a gorgeous prosthesis or cry over a discouraging prognosis. They share the good and the bad, bonded by common experience and solicitous understanding.

The four of us—all past 50—met in the comfortable atmosphere of the Rosewood Cafeteria in Porter Hospital, Denver, Colorado. It's a homey, tastefully decorated place. Windows stretch across the western view and the other two walls picture rolling hills and mountains spiked with trees in peaceful shades of cream, grey, warm beige and rosy mauve. Mahogany tables inlaid with a rose marbled pattern, upholstered chairs and booths invite patrons to relax.

Sarah, an elegant lady and piano teacher; Ann, a savvy, vivacious professional; Betty, a warm-hearted, motherly hospital employee, and I sat in a corner booth. They are attractive women working in the mainstream of life. The names are fictitious; the women are real.

After dinner I said, "My friend, Mary, who had a double mastectomy found that perfume resurrected her sense of womanhood after becoming flat chested for the second time since childhood. She had two attractive wigs, knew how to get the most out of makeup and dressed stylishly but perfume gave her the sense of still being female. What did it for you?"

Sarah   I use perfume every morning and twice again later in the day and I always wear earrings. I wasn't crazy about wigs. They felt like too much hair. Some of the girls have them thinned and styled. There are a lot of things you can do with them. Most of the time in our support group I have no clue as to who is wearing one and who isn't.

Ann   A good hairstyle did it for me. I don't feel comfortable if my hair is messed up. I worked while I was going through chemo and it sure helped. I don't want people to look at me and think "the poor thing." I want to look good...I want to look healthy.

Sarah   I used to wash my hair every morning but now I don't have the energy to do it that often. My hair is thinner as a result of the whole process and I think it's just that I'm getting old. I don't feel like putting on much makeup either. It's a subtle thing. I did want to look nice for the nurses and doctors in chemotherapy. It's part of my self-image. When I don't look nice, it doesn't feel good.

Ann   Appearance was important to me before the surgery. I do it for myself, so in that respect this wasn't a major change for me.

Sarah   I have spent a lot of time grieving and I'm not sure what that's about. I feel so ugly...you don't look ugly, you look like you, but I look in the mirror and say, "Oh, no." I think there is something about not having breasts that makes a woman feel ugly. It'll be five years since I was diagnosed and four years since the first surgery and then I had estrogen taken away from me which I think was a very aging thing. When I was taking it my skin was soft, I didn't have many wrinkles.

Betty   I'd die for estrogen...I loved it. I had an aunt who didn't have a wrinkle until she was 85. I'm lucky to have her good skin but it's drier than it was. It's always been dry but now it's dry dry.

Sarah   Doctors rarely give estrogen to women who have cancer. I don't believe we can take it with this kind of surgery.

Ann   I still have the image in here of me as a dumpy teenager and I can't get rid of it. When I was fortyish, I had half of my thyroid removed. When it was healing, the incision was bright red and so people would stare at it and I felt very self-conscious, very uncomfortable, seemed to detract from my looking okay. It doesn't bother me much any more but it certainly was difficult at the time. I had to shut off some of those negative feelings because there was nothing I could do about it...there it was and I couldn't cover it with a necklace.

Betty   Looking good has a lot to do with your well being.

Sarah   Well being has a lot to do with looking good. But it takes too much energy to shampoo every day and I had to push myself to put makeup on. I used to contour my blush and everything else but I had to cut makeup down to the absolute minimum. I know that sounds dumb but it takes a little longer than I wanted to stand there and do it.

Betty   When I didn't have to go to work, I didn't push. Sometimes it would take half a day to get to the point of putting on my makeup. I got into the habit of sewing before I got dressed.

Ann   Well, we all make choices along the way. There's a line we won't go over and have to say that's enough... that's all I can do. I have to push a little harder because I want to create an image I can be happy fitting into. This is the person I want to be. This is what it's going to take to do it even if I don't feel like getting there. I want that result because I'm more comfortable when I have it. I feel less vulnerable to the world, feel like I'm more the person I want to be. I sometimes think that the clothes and makeup I put on in the morning is my uniform. This is the way I wish to face the world, the way I want to be seen. It makes it easier for me to tackle the other things if I'm not worrying about how people perceive me.

Betty   You feel better when you're dressed well. When my mother was in a nursing home, they got everyone up and dressed regardless of what shape they were in. They reacted better when they were dressed.

Ann   You become the person you look like. Remember that song about whistling a happy tune whenever you feel afraid? You see the vision of what you want to be, you work to get it, and then you hope you fill it.

Sarah   You get this nice wonderful shell and hope you're big enough to be in it. One thing I've been doing is to create an outfit with jewelry and then write it down because I don't remember what goes with what. The only thing is that when I come to wear it, I may not feel like that outfit that day but at least it gives me something to start with.

Jo   I realize you're spooked by the ghost of death. In view of this, how do you empower yourself?

Ann   The more precious life becomes the more I want to live it fully. And looking good is part of it. I don't want to waste a minute looking ugly. When I realized I was going to go through something that would sap my energy, I prioritized. What's really important... what do I have to do as opposed to what can I let somebody else do? My personal appearance is mostly something only I can do. Yes, I can have a good hairdresser. Otherwise it's up to me. I mess around with my hair a lot, not as much as I used to though. Somebody else can clean my house. I look for ways to get things done easier so I have the time and energy to do things for my personal appearance.

Sarah   The thought of going out in public is enough to empower me. I won't go to the grocery store, anywhere, without fixing up. I'll stay at home and look pretty dumpy on the days I don't have the energy but when I have to go out, I will make some effort. It's not so much how people see me but what I see in the mirror.

Ann   When you look good, people tend to smile back at you, you get reinforcement from the world around you when you look nice and they are a mirror of sorts, I like that. I get reinforcement from people smiling at me, being pleasant.

Betty   I guess I get empowered by smiling. I've been accused of smiling too much but I get good reactions.

Sarah   You get yourself all fixed up and you look wonderful and then you have a drenching hot flash and your clothes and hair are damp and your face is bright red. Hot flashes are hard on self-esteem. It's disconcerting ... you forget where you are and what you're doing. It happens when you're under sudden stress. When I'm having a recital, getting up to speak, then I'm more likely to have one. I find activity brings it on, and if I get the tiniest bit too warm, then I have a hot flash, then I'm wet ... then cold. It can't last more than two minutes. I try to stop thinking about it. You *will* yourself to get through it. Maybe that's part of empowering.

Betty   When I'd go into a patient's room they'd look at my red face and ask, "Have you been out in the sun?" And, here I am having a hot flash. I had breast surgery at two separate times. The first time I had one breast removed. I went to this lingerie shop that specializes. It looks like Frederic's ... and they were very helpful. I tried on different sizes and different brands, trying to match up the breast I had left with a prosthesis. But when I had the other mastectomy, I bought skin supports. They stick on the skin and the other side is velcro where you put your breast form...no way will they fall off and you have no straps.

Sarah   Yes, you just put these strips of tape on the skin and then plop the boob on. I tried the tape once and didn't like it because I had a hard time getting them in the right place. But with a lowcut dress your breasts can look very natural with these skin supports. Just don't bend over!

Betty   The prostheses I have now I can wear in the bra or put them on the tape.

Ann   Clothes don't drape nicely for women if you don't have breasts. But some women won't wear prostheses.

Sarah   My friend won't.

Betty   I bought a lovely black lace bra for my prostheses. It's wonderful to wear. (to Jo) When we go to the rest room I'll show you what a prosthesis looks like. One of the girls in our group came in one evening with a sweat shirt on, lifted it up and said, "I want you all to know...here's my new breasts!"

Sarah   I have another story. I was so impressed with the prostheses of this beautiful woman I know that I wanted her to show them to my husband. So I asked her if she would and she said, "Sure." So she went out to the car with me and I introduced them and told him that she had agreed to show him her prostheses. So she did and said, "Here, feel it." He blushed timidly touched it and she said, "No, really feel it." The thing is she couldn't feel a thing. It doesn't ring any bells. Well, it rang his bells! And, then she plopped one out and said, "Hold it." Well, he's never gotten over it and gets a big laugh telling that story to his friends.

Betty   Having one breast was more difficult than none. Some women have both breasts removed if one has to go. I hated looking in the mirror when I just had the one...and to look down and see one lonely breast. I had some weird cells on the other side. They weren't cancerous but I didn't want to spend years wondering so I had it removed. I was never sorry. I'd rather be the way I am now. Being flat was much better that being lopsided. As soon as it was off I felt better. But at the time when I had my first mastectomy, nobody in the world could have talked me into having both removed. You're just concentrating on getting rid of the cancer, and health insurance won't pay for it just because you want it off.

Sarah   We grew up flat...flat we know, lopsided we don't. Having one breast reminds you of what you lost. The remaining breast was never a sex object. You think, "Well, at least I'll have one." But it doesn't work that way...it never came into play again. It was just this awful reminder.

Betty   Even if you told these things to a woman who was facing this choice, she wouldn't believe it. She'd still think she had to hang on to the one breast. You really have to live with it. So many people in our group have done the same thing. One had three biopsies in the other breast with the possibility of the cancer spreading and she would not let them do it, and she was in her 60s. We all look at things differently.

Ann   It isn't just your hair, it's your eyebrows, your eyelashes, your breasts...these are hard decisions.

Sarah   One woman said losing her hair was the hardest thing but she hadn't lost her breast and I don't know if she can still say that now that she's had a mastectomy.

Ann   Mine was caught early so I didn't go through that. They only took out some tissue. All I had was radiation after that.

Sarah   Some women say that reconstruction made them feel whole again but there's no feeling in them. It's totally aesthetic. Sometimes they have to be redesigned two or three times. Then, after all that, one might drop. Betty, have you ever seriously thought of breast reconstruction?

Betty   Not seriously...not for a minute actually. When I hear all the stories and how it hurts for a while, I don't want to go through that agony.

Sarah   A friend had it done. It's very complicated and controversial and with the right surgeon, can be very successful.

When we strive to heal mind and body, when we strive to keep the "candle of joy" burning brightly— and it takes lots of striving as these women have demonstrated, we can come out on the winning side.

Reconstructive Surgery. Recent developments and new procedures have made possible remarkable physical and psychological transformation through reconstructive breast surgery. The skill of the surgeon cannot be overemphasized. See Chapter 5 on *Erasing the Wrinkles* for guidelines in finding a qualified plastic surgeon. Breast reconstruction is a very emotional surgery. A woman needs a doctor who listens, treats her as an individual and who takes time to be attentive to her concerns.

Dr. Douglas McKinnon is a plastic and reconstructive surgeon, certified by the American Society of Plastic and Reconstructive Surgeons, Inc. Modern breast reconstruction goes back 15 years and Dr. McKinnon has been involved since that time. He says the choice for reconstruction after mastectomy is highly personal. Some women do well without it and do not wish to subject themselves to more surgery. Others want to look in the mirror and see their body as natural as possible. There are many different reliable procedures that meet their psychological and aesthetic expectations.

Dr. McKinnon advises that more often than not the operation is carried out in multiple stages and doesn't have to be complex or require lots of time off during recuperation. Reconstructions are different from their own breasts in feel and texture but even with minimal clothing they can look quite normal. Lots of women have had breast reconstruction and feel their body is whole again without the constant reminder of mastectomy.

Dr. McKinnon recommends that women facing mastectomy read *A Woman's Decision Breast Care, Treatment, and Reconstruction* by Karen Berger, a nurse, and John Bostwick III, M.D. It is enlightening even if reconstruction is not a consideration. The text is thorough, excellent, and easy-to-read, giving common sense answers to the apprehensions of women and to the questions of men who love their women and want to know how to intelligently help with decisions, how to play the role of supporting player, how to deal with sex and many other anxieties.

The Lingerie Solution. Every woman can find beautiful lingerie to fit her physical and emotional requirements. Women with single mastectomies can use their brassieres or any over- the-counter bra and insert a prosthesis in a cup or purchase a brassiere with a pocket for the prosthesis. (Prostheses look and feel amazingly life-like.) Pocket brassieres in many colors, styles and fabrics, even pretty laces, are also worn by women who have had bilateral mastectomies. These women may also choose the self-attachment prosthesis system. It contains adhesive supports that affix to the skin with velcro on the other side to hold the prostheses and can be worn with or without a bra as well as under swimsuits and strapless gowns.

Treva Stutzman, owner of Treva's, the biggest supplier of mastectomy products in Colorado, said that women who are shy, ashamed or reluctant can be assured of loving, understanding, sensitive guidance in lingerie shops like hers. They want to help clients find appropriate items that nurture their sense of well-being and their desire to be comfortable with how they look.

> **The face is the focal point of the appearance, not the torso, and the hair frames the face.**

Hair. There are hair products designed for women who are going through chemotherapy that promote healthy hair and scalp. With some combinations of chemotherapy drugs, hair loss is certain. When the doctor advises that it is, get a wig(s) before the process begins. (See pages 121, 122) Match it exactly to your hair or get an exciting change...blonde or red? But, only choose the shade(s) that complement your warm or cool skin undertones, and if necessary, have it styled to suit your taste. Some chapters of the American Cancer Society have "wig banks" that supply wigs at no charge. For additional information call 1-800-ACS-2345 or your local ACS chapter.

When the scalp gets hot or sensitive from wearing a wig, freshen with a mild shampoo to remove excess oil.

If hair loss is certain, you can have your eyes lined and brows permanent with cosmetic tattooing. Consider doing this before chemotherapy when nerves are stable. It is perfectly safe, will conserve your energy and gives you the comfort of knowing your face has this permanent enhancement. See **Cosmetic Tattooing** in Chapter 3, page 69.

Turbans and Scarves. When you don't want to wear a wig, you can wear turbans or scarves in cheerful, flattering colors. To soften the line around the forehead or cheeks, save hair from a cut and glue to a turban. Accessorize with pins and matching earrings. Turbans may be more user-friendly because it is sometimes difficult to raise the arms after surgery.

Skin care. Whatever your skin was, it will be dry and sensitive after chemotherapy. Even oily skin becomes dry. Check with your oncologist regarding exfoliators, masks, alpha hydroxy acid products, and retin A.

Cleansing. Use a gentle cleanser, not soap, that is formulated for dry skin. Cetaphil, Oilatum, and Aveeno Oilated Bar are dermatologist recommended.

Moisturizing. Moisturizers like Complex 15, Moisturel, Candermyl, Purpose Lotion, and Eucerin are indispensable. One that is too rich may cause breakouts. If it has a sun protection factor, that's even better. Moisturize the eye area as well but keep moisturizers and oils out of the eyes.

Sunscreen. Chemotherapeutic agents usually cause photosensitivity and an impaired immune system. Exposure to harmful UVA and UVB rays makes the skin vulnerable. A non- chemical sunscreen without strong chemicals[2] such as PABA or NON-PABA protects and prevents discolorations from getting darker. You also can get sun protection in moisturizers, lip balms, lipsticks and foundations.

Cosmetics. To avoid infection, throw away old makeup and start anew. Use cotton balls and disposable applicators. If you use brushes, cleanse weekly and soak in alcohol. Never share makeup, a good rule for all of us. Seeing how makeup magically transforms is fun. Beautifying your face is the bonus.

Concealant. Cancer treatments may change skin tone to sallow, ruddy or pale as well as cause hyper-pigmentation (dark spots). A quality concealant and foundation hide imperfections (see page 53). For puffiness under the eyes, put concealant into indentations around puffs, not on them. Use a concealer on spots, then apply foundation over entire face. If you put concealant on over foundation, get one the same shade. Lightly dust with translucent powder to set.

Foundation. A quality coverup foundation or base is an additional protection from the sun and adds flawless color to your face. Match it to the darkest tone in your complexion, a shade that revitalizes. Too light a shade will look chalky or ashy.

Defining the Eyes. The dark line created by lashes, not their length, is noticed most. The glue used for false lashes may be irritating especially if eyes feel dry and sensitive. There are fifteen shades of eye liners on the market. Select the one(s) that matches your skin tones best and define the upper and lower lids. Draw the line to about one-fourth of an inch from the inner corners. Do not close outer corners unless you have large eyes.

Brows. Brows are easily added or thickened by using either pencil or powder brow color. For the natural brow line, define three points on the browbone: the inner one over the inner eye corner, the mid-point over the pupil of the eye as you look straight into the mirror and the outer point. To find the outer point, take a pencil and hold it from edge of nose to outer corner of eye. The place where it touches the browbone is the outer point. (See page 57.) Connect these points by feathering in brow color, building it to natural-looking thickness. You can check an old photo for the best shape.

At any time, cosmetically tattooing brows and eye lining is an option that saves time and energy. See **Cosmetic Tattooing** on page 69.

Shadow. Use matte, fragrance free and non-drying eye shadows. Shades of brown flatter almost every eye color. See page pages 60 and 61 for enhancing techniques.

Cheeks. No brown or neutral colors. Select rose, mauve, terra-cotta, peach, or coral depending upon whether skin undertones are cool or warm. (Pages 71-73)

Lips. Lips may be very dry. Try this: 1. Apply lip balm with a SPF, let absorb; 2. Apply vaseline, let absorb; 3. Brush on an emollient lipstick. Procedure for applying lip color is: line lips to get the shape you want; fill in with lip color that blends with blush. (Page 73) *The least amount of product you use to get the best color, the longer it stays on.* A lip brush is an efficient tool for this and the best way to blend color into the lining.

Nails. For dry, brittle nails, use a cuticle conditioner and moisturizer to alleviate dehydration. (See page 139) If your oncologist approves, massage the cuticle area with an 8% alpha hydroxy acid product. Do not use nail wraps and never cut or push back cuticles because of possible infection. Do keep nails shaped. Be very cautious about buffing—as little as possible if at all.

Scent Sense. According to an ancient proverb, "Every perfume is a medicine." The perfumes, colognes and essences of today have progressed from being just pretty fragrances to their age-old mission of evoking relaxation, rejuvenation, well-being, even clarity of thought. As gentle as the breath of spring flowers, the ones we love quietly imitate part of our Self.

Ileostomy. Carol had ulcerative colitis. There was no known cause or cure, only total removal of the large intestine which necessitated an exterior opening in the abdomen and wearing an appliance. It changed her whole body image.

The years after the operation were very difficult. She was a closet ostomate (one who has an artificial passage for elimination), feeling like a freak, not wanting to talk about it to anyone including her family. It was like a horse on a coffee table. Everyone knows it's there but no one wants to say it is. "That was sick," Carol said. "A feeling of privacy is one thing but wanting to hide it or thinking I'm a freak is sick." She thought her children's friends would make fun of her. So, they pretended there were no problems.

Besides self-depreciation and the family's reluctance to discuss anything negative, she tried to cope with an alcoholic husband, whom she loved, depression, smoking, valium, self-medication, the whole unhappy cycle. She didn't know how to be open about her struggle. The closed family thinking kept her husband and children from talking about their worries, from sharing honest feelings... all part of the healing process for the whole family. "I could have helped them with their fears and they could have given me some strokes that I needed so badly. I didn't know how to allow their goodness to come to me," she said. No doctor ever suggested counseling and she thought it was crazy to go to a therapist.

After 19 years, at 48, Carol was shocked into reality when she verbally targeted her rage and helplessness at her husband. She committed herself for thirty days to a drug/alcohol treatment center. It was a spiritual quest as much as anything; she received the awakening she sought. "Getting this treatment was the biggest and best turning point in my life," she said. "I gave up valium cold turkey and smoking one year later."

Although it's still difficult to refer to her surgery and appliance, she no longer feels like a freak. She's divorced, but happier about herself than at any other time in her life. Both children are back living with her. They can talk about the bad stuff as well as the ever-growing good stuff. There are no longer any bad habits and if that horse ever shows up on the coffee table again, they're ready to talk about it. They don't have to pretend.

Carol feels that some kind of counseling to build self-appreciation is very important after surgical trauma especially if the patient has low self-esteem to begin with. As far as her appearance goes, the appliance doesn't show. There are no bulges. She wears a light panty girdle or control top panty-hose after checking with her doctor to be sure the pressure was okay. Both are comfortable. She wears anything but a bikini—even straight skirts and flat front jeans. A-line skirts and dresses look trimmer than gathers or pleats.

"We don't have to wear shapeless clothes like blouses hanging outside skirts or slacks. I find that looking the best I can is vitally important to my emotional health. We need that during and after recovery, and we need to fight depression. Looking our best is one way to do it."

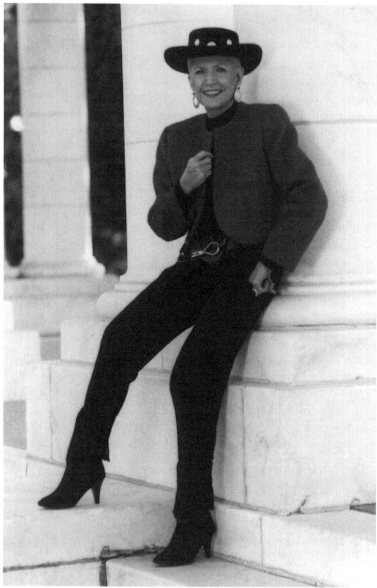

Betty Reed, a runway fashion model for over 40 years, has perfected the art of expressing the winning image through care, color and style. She has had two facelifts and may get another when she is 70. Diving and snorkeling in Mexico are her favorite sports. At 68, she passed the test to be a certified diver.

Epilogue

Birthdays Don't Count!

"The young are beautiful, but
the old are more beautiful
than the young."
—Walt Whitman,
Beautiful Women, 1860[1]

Why shouldn't personal beauty be part of longevity? More and more women realize that beauty is appropriate all our years, that this realization is regenerative and that it has little or no relevance to our birth date. So, why not develop a masterwork of individual style?

Suppose you are discouraged or just bored with the way you look, where do you begin? Start by tossing out the old stuff. Go through closets and drawers and give away or sell all jewelry, shoes, clothing that even hint of the matronly, dowdy or outmoded. If you haven't worn an item for two to three years, trash it. It's just taking up space. The same goes for cosmetics. Get rid of those you haven't worn. They do nothing for you, and instinctively you don't wear them. Make room for makeup with beautifying qualities, and fashions with zest as well as comfort.

Spend quiet time thinking about the new you. Release your imagination, and listen to your intuitive artistic sense. If you are in earnest, ideas will start percolating. Experiment with new techniques, new products, new colors. Feel the stimulus of getting out of that "old" rut! If we ever needed newness, it is now.

As we remove limitations, we have no idea what doors will open, what dreams will be realized. We "lose ourselves" in grandchildren, painting, music, gardening, career, romance, etc., but we find ourselves when we discover our individual specialness and the beauty potential that's been hiding behind old habits. A new career or enterprise, a new talent or hobby, enjoyable new friends, an exciting adventure, or unexpected opportunity are waiting for you when you are receptive to them. Your *nouvelle mode* facilitates the happening. This is not "pie in the sky," but you won't know for sure unless you try it, will you?

The way you dress expresses not only your personality but how you feel about yourself, and frequently, how you feel about other people. This personal style is influenced by:

A sense of appropriateness, a selectivity for what's best for you, individuality, comfort zone, style of living, and the occasion.

When you decide to put pizzazz into your appearance, give serious thought to the following concepts:

Don't dress according to a number. How often we get caught in that common mind trap, "I would love to wear that, but I'm just too old." Nonsense! Being over 50, 60, 70, or whatever the number doesn't mean we have to dress older. Our distinctive style and color personality still needs to be expressed. Forget the number. Instead, let what you wear say who you are.

In a wardrobe planning class a woman who was 26 said she was serious about her career, but was unhappy because people thought she was 18 and treated her as though she was. She wanted to look older. We encouraged her to dress, not "older," but more conservatively developing an individual sophistication that communicates maturity.

By contrast, consider my friend, Orra, who was pushing 70 but looking fiftyish. She appeared ageless. Petite with reddish-brown hair, she expressed an abundance of charisma and grace combined with disciplined professionalism. With her faultless application of makeup, simple but smart fashions, erect posture and congeniality, she was a true gentlewoman. For many years she owned and operated her own real estate agency and was the first woman to be elected president of the state board of realtors when she was almost 70. "Always look 10 to 20 years younger than you are," she counseled. She knew that appearance was a decisive factor in setting our stage for success...success in every avenue of life and especially in a competitive environment.

Donna Karan, fashion designer with The Donna Karan Company, New York City, said, "I don't think it [fashion and image] has anything to do with your age; I think it has to do with your state of mind. I see women in their fifties and sixties who are totally ageless...and look snazzy and... marvelous."[2]

Figure problems are not reasons to be unattractive. Beauty comes in all sizes and shapes. Fat or thin, short or tall does not determine our beauty potential, but self-thought does. Never forfeit the development of your stunning style to imperfections of the body. Accept the challenge to look your best and you will when you really want it.

The fashion industry designs for size 16 and over. By using compatible colors and couturier lines, as described in Chapter 8, we give balance to our profile. Dresses with large bold colorful prints give a striking look to the oversized woman as do slimming one-color suits.

Be dramatic with fashion when the occasion or your desire calls for it. Try striking combinations of color such as turquoise with fuchsia, fuchsia or red with yellow, coral with turquoise, or forest green with bright purple. The color plates in fashion magazines illustrate energizing color mixes.

If your legs are slender and pretty, wear the higher hems. For the petite figure, the leg-lengthening two-inch high heels are becoming and very feminine. Go for elegant, delicate, provocative and trend-setting fabrics and styles, if they are your forte and fit your comfort zone. Try the fun and flair of mixing the elegant with the casual, a lace or chiffon shirt with blue jeans, blue hose and matching pumps; a filmy chiffon shirt with a tailored or pleated skirt; a ribbed cashmere sweater worn over a brocade skirt. Experience the versatile Chanel jacket over shorts, long dresses, flippy skirts and even jeans. It's okay to break free of confining concepts—to wear sequins with the casual or sporty event, and sweaters for galas—if that suits your fancy. Listen to your intuition, and create pleasure-giving clothing combinations.

Liberate your personal sense of beauty. Convince yourself that you are getting better every day, not the opposite! Put forth your best, most colorful image in either the ethereal pastels, the vivid brights, rich deep tones, earthy hues, or striking monochromatic combos. Open your mind to that timeless, beautiful woman inside and let her out!

Be caring about yourself and you will see improvement in every aspect of your life. Some people think appearance is a very superficial aspect of our self. But, if you think about it, you realize that how you appear is a direct reflection of how you see yourself.

Once you've done your beauty work, forget the body and enjoy the flow of life. To constantly worry if your hair is right, if your lipstick is still on, if the slip is hanging or all the other ifs only adds another wrinkle. You checked everything, right? Now, forget it. Eliminate appearance anxiety. You're all right. To become an image addict, always checking for imperfections, is as bad as never doing it. Work with your inner artist, expand your self-awareness and stick like fly paper to your progress in beauty awareness.

Be discriminating about image advice. You are the ultimate expert. The guidelines throughout this book are just that—guides to achieving the image you want to impart. They are not inflexible. If you bend the basics and put together a smashing total statement that beckons compliments, but more important, makes you feel good, congratulate yourself.

The first point is perhaps the most important. The age number has little value when it comes to perceiving the attractive, timeless persona.

How to Find Your Best Overall Look

Your best look is a union of what's current and what's you. To develop the best look for women beyond their middle years, John Rund, International Guest Artist and Lecturer for Redken Laboratories, Inc., and Image Consultant in Denver, Colorado, suggests the following:

Being physically active contributes to looking your best. Diet, hygiene and attitude are more important the older we get.

Makeup

- To look naturally pretty, skin care is required.

- Be sure makeup base matches skin tone and avoid the shiny finish in foundation, powder or blush.

- Avoid frosted shades in eye shadow and lipstick. The satiny look of lip gloss is appropriate for evenings.

- Use grey or brown eye liner instead of black if you are Caucasian.

Hair

- Hair frames the face so the color needs to be soft and the style must flow. Afros and short perms with tight curls are aging.

- Find a hairdresser you can communicate with and ask what he/she specializes in. If it is cutting only, and you want coloring, perms and cuts, find a stylist who is an expert in all these areas. When you're ready for something different, collect photos of styles you like and discuss them with your hairdresser. One important consideration is: As your hair lightens, is it the right color for your complexion? The wrong one ages the face. Find out what your options are.

- Whoever said that all women over the magic five oh should wear short hair needs to spend a power lunch with Jackie Kennedy Onassis, Lauren Bacall, Barbara Walters, or Sophia Loren. If you like short hair, fine; if you don't, refuse to be influenced. Wear it longer.

Fashion

- Be willing to take the time to look like yourself—only better. Be the best you! Keeping up with style is keeping up with you, and if you're doing that, you're looking younger. Move with the times!

- Accentuate your best features; bring attention to them. Don't concentrate on negative ones.

- Get in touch with your personal style. If you are unsure about it, find an image consultant and build a relationship based on how you want to look.

- Wear color. Black and white can be harsh.

- Add glamour to your appearance. Don't be afraid of being dramatic or adding a splash of whimsy such as a rakish scarf or red high top tennis shoes! Put distinctive items in your wardrobe.

- Feel comfortable in everything you wear and dare to experiment.

The purpose of makeup and fashion is not to create a stylized mannikin. It is to depict the beauty of the person you are.

Isn't "panache" a wonderful word? Perhaps "flair" or dash" are the closest English synonyms to this fascinating French adjective. What a lift to the spirit to have at least one outfit that has panache! When you have one, look for another.

Although high fashion garments are exhilarating, shrewd shoppers manage to dress supremely chic using good budget sense and all discount and sales options. Constancy in taste is possible at any price level. Interchangeable and coordinating outfits offer multiple choices with economy. We don't need lots of clothes when we have mixables.

I seldom see the husbands of clients, but I did meet two whose wives were surprisingly similar. Harriet is in her mid-50s and Susan, just over 60. Both have been married for 30 or more years, and it was obvious their spouses still admire them. These women have cheerful dispositions with sunny smiles, a zest for life and pride in appearance—on a modest budget—that is not the least bit egotistic.

This does not suggest that beauty-consciousness is the solution to matrimonial bliss. Far from it! But, for centuries women have known they must nurture appearance with more care than men do. No woman knew this more than Queen Elizabeth I of England, who during her reign in the 1500s wanted to impress, influence, be remembered and loved by her people. She portrayed herself as a caring monarch in appearance as much as anything, and it was no accident. She planned it that way and wanted it that way up to her last breath. Many modern women who are over fifty and very visible in the media and public life are repeating the same philosophy.

Putting our best look forward is essential to squeezing every ounce of satisfaction out of life. Being a lovely presence adds pleasure to our world, just as the fragrance of each blossom from the delicate wild flower to the exquisite rose whispers a note of joy to the beholder.

What message do you get
When you contemplate
A lovely little flower?
Be like me,
Make beauty a part of your life.

Leonard Andrews
New York Daily News[3]

Catherine Ponder in *The Prospering Power of Love*[4] tells of a way to create beauty, "You can glorify your own appearance...by creating as much beauty as possible.

"A famous actress was once asked how she stayed so young, though she was actually past 70. Her reply was that she remained youthful by looking at beauty, appreciating beauty, thinking about beauty.

"You can have more beauty in your world if you will begin right where you are to add whatever touches of beauty are possible. As you do this, beauty will multiply in your life. As you dwell more and more on beauty and do all that is possible to produce it in your world, you will become more successful and prosperous."

Katherine Hepburn[5] said she was glad to be born a woman. "I think women are nicer. Don't you?" Think of all the parts they play in one lifetime—child, lover, mother, wife, grandmother, comforter, confidante, teacher, clubwoman, volunteer, provider, church member, homemaker, storekeeper, businesswoman, artist, professional. The list goes on and on. While filling many roles simultaneously, women endure unbelievable hardships that would stymie many a stalwart male, yet they keep plugging along, often forgetting their own needs in favor of another's.

So, it's right to appreciate ourselves, to view ourselves compassionately, not critically. Self-depreciation accomplishes nothing. Passing middle age is a signal for new beginnings and happenings. If bulges or wrinkles can't be corrected, so what? Stop worrying about them. It's okay to have wrinkles and bulges. They're part of growing up! Beauty has many faces and forms. Youth is one; maturity is another with deeper meaning and the potential to rival youth. The youth ethic is okay, but the ageless ethic is better.

Many times we look better than we realize. We have a bad habit of listening to a personalized putdown syndrome. As I was waiting to interview a doctor for this book, I talked to his receptionist. Her silver-grey hair was smoothly coiffed and framed an openly friendly face with soft makeup colorings. She wore a two-piece grey knit suit flecked with green and turquoise that typified not age or youth but timeless style. When I told her she looked lovely, she exclaimed with genuine surprise, "Oh my, do I really?" Then she stood up and said, "But, just look at how fat I am!" She thought a little plumpness around the middle was a detraction. Actually, I never got down to her waistline. It didn't matter.

Living longer, actively and healthier is the trend of this era, and how we define appearance as well as the way we spend our time is important. In this context, birthdays don't count.

Denouncing limiting self-talk, often caused by the critical tapes that creep in from a judgmental society, is not enough. We must cultivate the viewpoint of positive expectancy, automatically questioning the legitimacy of the negative. It takes mental strength to exercise this wisdom, but the result is a contented and rewarding experience.

And, oh yes, SMILE. The loveliest you shines through the window of your smile. It's the best advertisement for the person you are and your passport to receiving more of what's rightfully yours—continuing happiness and fulfillment.

P

Notes

Introduction

[1]Maltz, Dr. Maxwell, *Psycho-Cybernetics*, Englewood Cliffs, NY: Prentice Hall, a division of Simon & Schuster, 1960, 1988

[2]Pickford, Kaylan, *Always Beautiful*, NY: G.P. Putnam's Sons, 1985

[3]Davis, Julie, *The Allure Book*, New York: Bantam Books, 1984, p. 8

Chapter 1
The Magic of Color

[1]Marshall Editions Ltd. of London, *Color*, Los Angeles: The Knapp Press, 1980. p. 10

[2]Itten, Johannes, *The Art of Color*, London: Van Norstrand Reinhold Co., 1973, p. 16

[3]Birren, Faber, Color *Psychology and Color Therapy*, Secaus, NJ: Citadel Press, 1961

[4]Gerson, Joel, *Standard Book for Professional Estheticians*, Bronx, NY: Milady Publishing Corp., 1984, p. 204

[5]*Ibid.*

Chapter 2
The Basics

[1]Kerr, Jean, "Mirror, Mirror on the Wall, I Don't Want to Hear One Word Out of You," in *The Snake Has All the Lines*, 1960

[2]Wesley-Hosford, Zia, *Face Value*, NY: Bantam Books, 1986, p. 36

[3]*Ibid.*, p. 10

[4]Gerson, Joel, Standard Book for *Professional Estheticians*, Bronx, NY: Milady Publishing Corp., 1984, p. 204

[5]Alexander, Dale, *Dry Skin and Common Sense*, West Hartford, CT: Witkower Press, Inc., 1978

[6]Schrader, Constance, *No More Wrinkles*, NY: Signet-New American Library, 1986.

[7]Reilly, Harold J. and Ruth Hagy Brod, *The Edgar Cayce Handbook for Health*, Virginia Beach, VA: A.R.E. Press, 1975

[8]*Ibid.*

[9]Ray, Tony, Angela Hynes, *The Silver/Grey Beauty Book*, New York: Rawson Associates, 1987.

[10]Carnegie, Dale, *How to Win Friends and Influence People*, New York: Pocket Books, 1982

[11]Landers, Ann, *Gems*, Chicago: 1988

[12]Lawson, Donna, *Prevention's Guide to Looking Fit and Fabulous at 40*, Emmaus, PA: Rodale Press, 1987

[13]University of California, Berkeley *Wellness Letter*, June 1989

[14]Brown, Michele and Anne O'Connor, *Hammer and Tongues*, NY: St. Martin's Press, Inc.

[15]*Vogue Magazine*, October 1986 (Fitzpatrick)

[16]Gerson, *Standard Book for Professional Estheticians*, p. 204

[17]Bruce, Jeffrey, Sherry Cohen, *About Face*, New York, NY: Putnam Publishing Group, 1984, p. 130

[18]Linda Fang, M.D. is one of the first clinical dermatologists to put a non-chemical sunscreen into moisturizers and foundations.

Chapter 3
Be Your Own Makeup Artist

[1]Rubinstein, Helena, *My Life For Beauty*, NY: Simon & Schuster, 1966

[2]Bruce, Jeffrey, Sherry Cohen, *About Face*, New York, NY: Putnam Publishing Group, 1984, p. 129

[3]*Ibid.*, p. 129

[4]Davis, Julie, *The Allure Book*, New York: Bantam Books, 1984, p. 94

[5]Vaughan-Richards, Ayo, *Black and Beautiful*, London, UK: Collins, 1986

[6]*Ibid.*

[7]*Porter Hospital Newspaper*, Denver, CO, Spring 1987

Chapter 4
You Can Brighten Your Smile

[1]Viorst, Judith, *Forever Fifty,* New York, NY: Simon and Schuster, 1989, p. 49
[2]*Modern Maturity,* "Braces—At My Age?" October-September 1987, p. 27
[3]*Senior World/Los Angeles,* CA, May 1990

Chapter 5
Erasing the Wrinkles

[1]*Senior Spotlight,* Denver, CO, April 1989, p. 15
[2]Maltz, Dr. Maxwell, *Psycho-Cybernetics,* Englewood Cliffs, NJ: Prentice Hall, a division of Simon & Schuster, 1960, 1988
[3]Alexander, *Dry Skin and Common Sense*
[4]Jacobson, Carlotta Karlson, *How to be Wrinkle-Free,* NY: Putnam Publishing Group, 1986
[5]Federal Trade Commission, Office of Consumer/Business Education, *Facts for Consumers, Cosmetic Surgery,* Washington, D.C., March 1990
[6]Maltz, *Pscho-Cybernetics,* p. 152.

Chapter 6
Hair

[1]Jacobson, *How to be Wrinkle-Free*
[2]Robertson, Laurel, Carol Flinders, Bronwen Godfrey, *Laurel's Kitchen,* Petaluma, CA: Bantam/Nilgiri Press, 1978
[3]Wesley-Hosford, *Face Value*
[4]*Bazaar* magazine, August 1990, p. 124

Chapter 7
Fashion for Your Figure

[1]Weiland, Barbara and Leslie Wood, *Clothes Sense,* Portland, OR: Palmer/Pletsch Associates, 1984.

Chapter 8
Hands

[1]Bozic, Patricia, *30 Days to Beautiful Nails*, NY: Warner Books, 1984, p. 64.

[2]Arpel, Adrien, *851 Fast Beauty Fixes and Facts*, NY: Dell Publishing Co., 1985, p. 152

[3]Bozic, *30 Days to Beautiful Nails*, pp. 11, 18.

Chapter 9
Accessories

[1]Nelson, LeAnn L., *Accessories ... What a Finish!*, Denver, CO: 1988

[2]*Senior Focus*, Bremerton, WA, December 1990

[3]Norman, Scot, *How to Buy Great Shoes*, New York, NY: Crown Publishers, 1988

Chapter 10
Coping With Defeminizing Surgery

[1]Mulberry Hill Press 1-800-294-4714

[2]One non-chemical, inert ingredient is titanium dioxide, used as a physical barrier to block a broad spectrum of UV radiation. The Linda Sý Non-Chemical Sunscreen SPF 16 is available from dermatologists or call 1-800-232-3376 in California and 1-800-422-3376 outside California.

Epilogue
Birthdays Don't Count!

[1]Whitman, Walt, *Leaves of Grass*

[2]*Vogue*, June 1987

[3]*Newsweek*, August 18, 1986

[4]Ponder, Catherine, *The Prospering Power of Love*, Marina Del Rey, CA: Devorss and Company, 1983, p. 64

[5]*Ladies Home Journal*, October 1987

Bibliography

Alexander, Dale, *Dry Skin and Common Sense*, West Hartford, CT: Witkower Press, Inc., 1978

Arpel, Adrien, *851 Fast Beauty Fixes and Facts*, NY: Dell Publishing Co., 1985

Berger, Karen and John Bostwick III, M.D., *A Woman's Decision Breast Care, Treatment, and Reconstruction*, NY: The C. V. Mosby Company, 1994

Birren, Faber, *Color Psychology and Color Therapy*, Secaus, NJ: Citadel Press, 1961

Boughton, Patricia and Mary Ellen Hughes, *The Buyer's Guide to Cosmetics*, NY: Random House 1981

Bozic, Patricia, *30 Days to Beautiful Nails*, NY: Warner Books, 1984

Brown, Michele and Anne O'Connor, *Hammer and Tongues*, NY: St. Martin's Press, Inc.

Bruce, Jeffrey, Sherry Cohen, *About Face*, New York, NY: G.P. Putnam's Sons, 1984

Carnegie, Dale, *How to Win Friends and Influence People*, New York: Pocket Books, 1982

Davis, Julie, *The Allure Book*, New York: Bantam Books, 1984

Feder, M.D., Lewis M. and Jane MacLean Craig, *About Face*, New York, NY: Warner Books, 1984

Gerson, Joel, *Standard Book for Professional Estheticians*, Bronx, NY: Milady Publishing Corp., 1984

Hill, Napoleon, *The Law of Success*, Chicago, IL: Success Unlimited, Inc., 1979

Hjelmsted, Lois Tschetter, *Fine Black Lines*, Denver, CO: Mulberry Hill Press, 1993

Itten, Johannes, *The Art of Color*, London: Van Norstrand Reinhold Co., 1937

Jackson, Carole, *Color Me Beautiful*, New York: Ballantine Books, 1981

Jacobson, Carlotta Karlson, *How to Be Wrinkle-Free*, New York: G. P. Putnam's Sons, 1986

Kentner, Bernice, *Tie Me Up With Rainbows*, Concord, CA: Kenkra Publishers, 1980

Lawson, Donna, *Prevention's Guide to Looking Fit and Fabulous at 40*, Emmaus, PA: Rodale Press, 1987

Maltz, Dr. Maxwell, *Psycho-Cybernetics*, NY: Simon & Schuster, 1960

Marshal Editions Ltd. of London, *Color*, *Los Angeles:* The Knapp Press, 1980

Morris, Edwin T., *Fragrance*, New York: Charles Scribner's Sons, 1984

Novid, Dr. Nelson Lee, *Saving Face*, New York: Franklin Watts, 1986

Pickford, Kaylan, *Always Beautiful*, NY: G.P. Putnam's Sons, 1985

Ponder, Catherine, *The Prospering Power of Love*, Marina Del Rey, CA: Devorss and Company, 1983

Ray, Tony, Angely Hynes, *The Silver/Grey Beauty Book*, New York: Rawson Associates, 1987

Reilly, Harold J. and Ruth Hagy Brod, *The Edgar Cayce Handbook for Health*, Virginia Beach, VA: A.R.E. Press, 1975

Robertson, Laurel, Carol Flinders, Bronwen Godfrey, *Laurel's Kitchen*, CA: Bantam/Nilgiri Press, 1978

Schrader, Constance, *No More Wrinkles*, NY: Signet-New American Library, 1986

Stone, Justin F., *T'ai Chi Chih!*, San Luis Obispo, CA: Satori Resources, 1987

Straley, Carol, *Sensational Scarfs*, NY: Crown Publishers, Inc., 1985

Vaughan-Richards, Ayo, *Black and Beautiful*, London, UK: Collins, 1986

Viorst, Judith, *Forever Fifty*, NY, NY: Simon and Schuster, 1989.

Weiland, Barbara and Leslie Wood, *Clothes Sense*, Portland, OR: Palmer/Pletsch Associates, 1984

Wesley-Hosford, Zia, *Face Value*, NY: Bantam Books, 1986

Index

Order Form

IF YOU WANT TO GIVE A BOOK
TO A FRIEND OR RELATIVE, CONSIDER

Look Like A Winner After 50
With Care, Color and Style.................................$15.95

Make check or money order payable to
Golden Aspen Publishing, P.O. Box 370333,
Denver, CO 80237-0333.

Sales Tax for Colorado residents only
Please add $1.15 sales tax for each book shipped to a Denver County address;
outside Denver County, add 48 cents for each book.

Shipping
Book rate: $2.00 for first book, 80 cents for each additional one. Delivery may
take three to four weeks.

I am enclosing $ _____ for _____ book(s).

NAME _____

ADDRESS _____

CITY/STATE/ZIP _____

PHONE (_____) _____

Satisfaction Guaranteed!
If for any reason you are not completely satisfied,
simply return your purchase to us within 30 days, and
we'll promptly refund the full amount.

Thank you for your order.

QUANTITY ORDERS INVITED
For discount on quantity orders,
call (303) 694-6555